For
John —
My beautiful
I love you —
Namaste —
Michelle

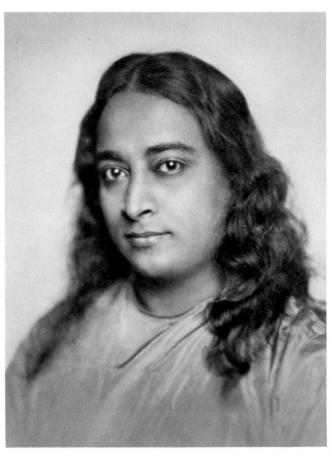

Paramahansa Yogananda

Sayings
of
Paramahansa Yogananda

SELF-REALIZATION FELLOWSHIP
Founded by Paramahansa Yogananda

SAYINGS OF PARAMAHANSA YOGANANDA
(Formerly "The Master Said")

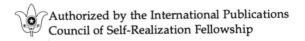

Authorized by the International Publications Council of Self-Realization Fellowship

Self-Realization Fellowship was founded in 1920 by Paramahansa Yogananda to serve as the channel for worldwide dissemination of his teachings.

Library of Congress Catalog Card Number: 79–66287
ISBN 0–87612–115–6
Printed in the United States of America
10651–54321

CONTENTS

ILLUSTRATIONS

Paramahansa Yogananda:

facing page

Other:

PUBLISHER'S NOTE

Since Paramahansa Yogananda's *Autobiography of a Yogi* was first published in 1946, his writings have received recognition in all parts of the world—from the literary and general public as well as from his followers. It is therefore not surprising that there are now a number of other publishers, organizations, and individuals claiming to represent his teachings. Some are borrowing the name of this beloved world teacher to further their own societies or interests, or to gain recognition for themselves. Others are presenting what is purported to be his "original" teachings, but what is in fact material taken from publications that had been poorly edited by temporary helpers or compiled from incomplete notes taken during Paramahansa Yogananda's classes. The Guru was very dissatisfied with the presentation of this material, and later did much work on it and gave specific instructions for its correction and clarification.

Readers sometimes inquire how they can be sure that a publication accurately presents the life and teachings of Sri Yogananda. In response to these inquiries, we would like to explain that Paramahansa Yogananda founded Self-Realization Fellowship in 1920 to be the instrument for worldwide dissemination of his teachings. He personally chose and trained those close disciples who constitute the Self-Realization Fellowship Publications Council, giving them specific guidelines for the publishing of his writings, lectures, and *Self-Realization Lessons*. The presence in a publication of the emblem shown above, or the statement, "Authorized by the International Publications Council of Self-Realization Fellowship," assures the reader of the authenticity of that work.

SELF-REALIZATION FELLOWSHIP

FOREWORD

Who may justly be called a master? No ordinary person, surely, is worthy of this title. And but rarely does there appear on earth one of that holy company to whom the Galilean master referred: "He that believeth on me [the Christ Consciousness], the works that I do shall he do also."*

Men become masters through discipline of the little self, or ego; through elimination of all desires save one — the desire for God; through singlehearted devotion to Him; and through deep meditation, or soul communion with the Universal Spirit. He whose consciousness is unshakably established in the Lord, the sole Reality, may rightfully be called a master.

Paramahansa Yogananda, the master whose words are lovingly recorded in this book, was a world teacher. Pointing out the essential unity of all great scriptures, he strove to unite East and West in the lasting ties of spiritual understanding. Through his life and writings he ignited in innumerable hearts a divine spark of love for God. He lived fearlessly by the highest precepts of religion; and proclaimed that all devotees of the Heavenly Father, no matter what their creeds, are equally dear to Him.

* John 14:12.

A college education and many years of spiritual training in his native land, India, under the Spartan discipline of his guru (spiritual teacher), Swami Sri Yukteswar, prepared Paramahansa Yogananda for his mission in the West. He came to Boston in 1920 as the Indian delegate to a Congress of Religious Liberals, and remained in America for over thirty years (except for a return visit to India in 1935–36).

Phenomenal success attended his efforts to awaken in others a desire for attunement with God. In hundreds of cities his yoga* classes broke all attendance records. He personally initiated in yoga 100,000 students.

For devotees who desire to follow the monastic path, the Master founded several Self-Realization Fellowship ashram centers in southern California. There many truth seekers study, work, and engage in meditational practices that quiet the mind and awaken soul awareness.

The following incident in the Master's life in America illustrates the loving reception given him by men endowed with spiritual perception:

On a tour of various parts of the United States, he stopped one day to visit a Christian monastery. The brothers received him with some apprehension, noting his dark skin, long black hair, and ocher robe—traditional garb of monks of the Swami Order.* Thinking him a heathen,

* See glossary.

they were about to refuse him an audience with the abbot, when that good man entered the room. With beaming face and open arms, he approached and embraced Paramahansaji*, exclaiming, "Man of God! I am happy you have come."

This book reveals other personal glimpses of the Master's myriad-faceted nature, gleaming with compassionate understanding of man and boundless love for God.

It is a privilege and a sacred trust for Self-Realization Fellowship, the society founded by Paramahansa Yogananda for the dissemination and perpetuation of all his teachings and writings, to publish this selection of sayings of the Master. This volume is dedicated to his worldwide family of Self-Realization Fellowship students, and to all other seekers of truth.

* See "ji" in glossary.

SAYINGS OF
PARAMAHANSA YOGANANDA

Sayings of
Paramahansa Yogananda

"Sir, what should I do to find God?" a student asked. The Master said:

"During every little period of leisure, plunge your mind into the infinite thought of Him. Talk to Him intimately; He is the nearest of the near, the dearest of the dear. Love Him as a miser loves money, as an ardent man loves his sweetheart, as a drowning person loves breath. When you yearn for God with intensity, He will come to you."

• • •

A student complained to the Master that he could find no work. The Guru* said:

"Do not hold that destructive thought. As a part of the universe, you have an essential place in it. If necessary, shake up the world to find your work! Don't give up and you will succeed."

* See glossary.

"I wish I had faith, Master," a man said. Paramahansaji replied:

"Faith has to be cultivated, or rather uncovered within us. It is there but has to be brought out. If you watch your life you will see the innumerable ways in which God works through it; your faith will thus be strengthened. Few people look for His hidden hand. Most men consider the course of events as natural and inevitable. They little know what radical changes are possible through prayer!"

•   •   •

A certain disciple took offense at any mention of her faults. One day Paramahansaji said:

"Why should you object to being corrected? Is that not what I am here for? My guru often censured me in front of others. I didn't resent it because I knew Sri Yukteswarji was trying to banish my ignorance. I am not sensitive about criticism now; no diseased spots remain in me to be hurt by anyone's touches.

"That is why I tell you plainly about your defects. If you do not heal the sore places in your mind, you will wince every time that others rub them."

•   •   •

The Master said to a group of disciples:

"The Lord has arranged for us this visit to

the earth, but most of us become undesirable guests by considering certain things here as our very own. Forgetting the temporary nature of our stay, we form various attachments: 'my home,' 'my work,' 'my money,' 'my family.'

"But when our earth-visa expires, all human ties vanish. We are forced to leave behind us all we had thought we possessed. The only One who accompanies us everywhere is our Eternal Relative, God.

"Realize *now* that you are the soul and not the body. Why wait for Death rudely to instruct you?"

. . .

The Master had found it necessary to scold a disciple about a serious error. Later he said with a sigh:

"I wish to influence others only by love. I just wilt when I am forced to train them in other ways."

. . .

An arrogant intellectual, discussing complicated philosophical problems, sought to confuse the Master. Paramahansaji said, smiling:

"Truth is never afraid of questions."

"I am too deeply enmeshed in mistakes to make any spiritual progress," a student confided sadly to Paramahansaji. "My bad habits are so strong that I am worn out by my efforts to fight them."

"Shall you be better able to fight them tomorrow than today?" the Master asked. "Why add today's mistakes to yesterday's? You have to turn to God some time, so isn't it better to do it now? Just give yourself to Him and say: 'Lord, naughty or good, I am Your child. You must take care of me.' If you keep on trying, you will improve. 'A saint is a sinner who never gave up.'"

• • •

"In the absence of inward joy, men turn to evil," the Master said. "Meditation on the God of Bliss permeates us with goodness."

• • •

"Body, mind, and soul are interrelated," the Master said. "You have a duty to the body — keeping it fit; a duty to the mind—developing its powers; and a duty to the soul—daily meditation on the Source of your being. If you fulfill your duty to the soul, body and mind will benefit, too; but if you neglect the soul, eventually body and mind also will suffer."

"Everything in creation has individuality," the Master said. "The Lord never repeats Himself. Similarly, in man's divine search there are infinite variations of approach and expression. The romance of each devotee with God is unique."

• • •

"Does your training help students to be at peace with themselves?" a visitor inquired. Paramahansaji answered:

"Yes, but that is not my central teaching. It is best to be at peace with God."

• • •

A visitor to the hermitage expressed doubt about man's immortality. The Master said:

"Try to realize you are a divine traveler. You are here for only a little while, then depart for a dissimilar and fascinating world.* Do not limit your thought to one brief life and one small earth. Remember the vastness of the Spirit that dwells within you."

• • •

"Man and Nature are indissolubly linked and bound in a common fate," the Master said. "The

* See "astral worlds" in glossary.

forces of Nature work together to serve man—the sun, the earth, the wind, the rain aid in producing his food. Man guides Nature, though usually unknowingly. Floods, tornadoes, earthquakes, and all other natural calamities are results of multitudinous wrong human thoughts. Each wayside flower is an expression of someone's smile, each mosquito an embodiment of someone's biting speech.

"The servant Nature rebels and grows unruly when the master of creation sleeps. The more spiritually awakened he becomes, the more easily shall he control Nature."

• • •

"Milk poured into water mixes with it; but butter, churned from milk, floats on top of water," the Master said. "Similarly, the milk of an ordinary person's mind is quickly diluted by the waters of delusion.* The man of spiritual self-discipline churns the milk of his mind into the butter-state of divine stability. Free from earthly desires and attachments, he is able to float serenely on the waters of worldly life, ever intent on God."

* See "maya" in glossary.

When a certain student became sick, Paramahansaji advised her to see a doctor. A disciple asked:

"Master, why didn't *you* heal her?"

"Those who have received from God the power of healing use it only when He so commands," the Guru replied. "The Lord knows that sometimes it is necessary for His children to undergo suffering. Men who want divine healings should be ready to live in accordance with God's laws. No permanent healing is possible if a person continues to make the same mistakes and thus invites the return of the disease.

"True healing is effected only through spiritual understanding," he went on. "Man's ignorance of his real nature or soul is the root cause of all other evils—physical, material, and mental."

. . .

"Sir, I do not seem to be progressing in my meditations. I see and hear nothing," a student said. The Master replied:

"Seek God for His own sake. The highest perception is to feel Him as Bliss, welling up from your infinite depths. Don't yearn for visions, spiritual phenomena, or thrilling experiences. The path to the Divine is not a circus!"

"The whole universe is made of Spirit," the Master said to a group of disciples. "A star, a stone, a tree, and a man are equally composed of the Sole Substance, God. To bring into being a diversified creation, the Lord had to bestow on everything the *appearance* of individuality.

"We would quickly tire of the earthly spectacle if we could easily see that only One Person is producing the play — writing the script, painting the scenery, directing the cast, acting all parts. But 'the show must go on'; therefore the Master Dramatist has manifested throughout the cosmos an inconceivable ingenuity and an inexhaustible variety. To unrealities He has given a seeming reality."

"Master, why must the show go on?" a disciple inquired.

"It is God's *lila,* play or sport," the Guru answered. "He has a right to separate Himself into many, if He so chooses. The point of it all is for man to see through His trick. If God did not cover Himself with the veils of *maya,* there could be no Cosmic Game of creation. We are permitted to play hide-and-seek with Him, trying to find Him and win the Grand Prize."

•   •   •

To a group of disciples the Master said:
"I know that if I had nothing, in you all I

possess friends who would do everything for me. And you know that in me you possess a friend who will help you in every way. We are looking at God in one another. It is the most beautiful relationship."

. . .

The Master usually insisted on silence among those around him. He explained: "From the depths of silence the geyser of God's bliss shoots up unfailingly and flows over man's being."

. . .

Disciples deemed it a privilege to render service to the Guru, who labored unceasingly for their welfare. To a group of devotees who had done some work for him, the Master said:

"You are all so kind to me with your many attentions."

"O no! It is you who are kind to us, Master," a disciple exclaimed.

"God is helping God," Paramahansaji said with his sweet smile. "That is the 'plot' of His drama of human life."

"Destroy all desire; get rid of the ego—all this sounds very negative to me, Master," a student remarked. "Abandoning so much, what shall I have left?"

"Everything, really, because you shall be wealthy in Spirit, the Universal Substance," the Master replied. "No longer a bewildered beggar, content with a crust of bread and a few bodily comforts, you shall have regained your sublime place as a son of the Infinite Father. That is not a negative state!"

He added, "Banishing the ego allows the true Self to shine forth. Divine realization is a state impossible to explain, because nothing else can be compared to it."

•   •   •

Explaining the Trinity to a group of disciples, the Master used this simile:

"We may say that God the Father, existing in the vibrationless void beyond phenomena, is the Capital that 'backs' creation. The Son, or intelligent Christ Consciousness that permeates the universe, is Management. And the Holy Ghost, or divine invisible vibratory power that produces all forms in the cosmos, is Labor."*

* See "Sat-Tat-Aum" in glossary.

"Master, you have taught us not to pray for things, but to desire only that God reveal Himself to us. Should we never ask Him to supply a particular need?" a disciple inquired.

"It is not wrong to tell the Lord that we want something," Paramahansaji replied, "but it shows greater faith if we simply say: 'Heavenly Father, I know that Thou dost anticipate my every need. Sustain me according to Thy will.'

"If a man is eager to own a car, for instance, and prays for it with sufficient intensity, he will receive it. But possession of a car may not be the best thing for him. Sometimes the Lord denies our little prayers because He intends to bestow on us a better gift." He added, "Trust more in God. Believe that He who created you will maintain you."

•　•　•

A disciple who felt that he had failed in a difficult spiritual test was reviling himself. The Master said:

"Do not think of yourself as a sinner. To do so is a desecration of the divine image within you. Why identify yourself with your weaknesses? Instead, affirm the truth: *I am a child of God.* Pray to Him: 'Naughty or good, I am Thine own. Reawaken my memory of Thee, O Heavenly Father!'"

"I often think that God forgets man," commented a visitor to the Encinitas* Hermitage. "The Lord certainly keeps His distance."

"It is man who keeps his distance," the Master replied. "Who seeks God? The mental temples of most persons are filled with idols of restless thoughts and desires; the Lord is ignored. Even so, from time to time He sends His enlightened sons to remind man of his divine heritage.

"God never forsakes us. Silently He works in every way to help His beloved children and to hasten their spiritual progress."

• • •

To a young devotee seeking his advice, the Master said:

"The world creates bad habits in you, but the world will not stand responsible for your mistakes springing from those habits. Then why give all your time to a false friend—the world? Reserve an hour a day for scientific soul exploration. Doesn't the Lord—the Giver of your life, your family, your money, and everything else — deserve one twenty-fourth part of your time?"

* Encinitas is a small seaside town in southern California. It is the site of an SRF Ashram Center founded by Yoganandaji in 1937.

"Sir, why do some persons ridicule saints?" a disciple asked. The Master replied:

"Evildoers hate the truth, and worldly people are satisfied with the ups and downs of life. Neither want to change; the thought of a saint therefore makes them uncomfortable. They may be compared to a man who has lived for many years in a dark room. Someone comes and switches on the light. To the half-blind man the sudden brilliance seems unnatural."

•   •   •

Speaking one day about racial prejudice, the Master said, "God is not pleased to be insulted when He wears His dark suits."

•   •   •

"We should neither be frightened by nightmares of pain nor unduly elated by dreams of beautiful experiences," the Master said. "By dwelling on these inevitable dualities or 'pairs of opposites' of *maya*, we lose the thought of God, the Changeless Abode of Bliss. When we awaken in Him we shall realize that mortal life is only a picture made of shadows and light, cast on a cosmic movie screen."

"Though I try to calm my mind, I lack the power to banish restless thoughts and to penetrate the world within," a visitor remarked. "I must be lacking in devotion."

"Sitting in the silence trying to feel devotion may often get you nowhere," the Master said. "That is why I teach scientific techniques of meditation. Practice them and you will be able to disconnect the mind from sensory distractions and from the otherwise ceaseless flow of thoughts."

He added, "By *Kriya Yoga** one's consciousness functions on a higher plane; devotion to the Infinite Spirit then arises spontaneously in man's heart."

•   •   •

Sri Yoganandaji described as follows the state of "inaction" mentioned in the Bhagavad-Gita:†

"When a true yogi performs an action, karmically it is like writing on water. No mark remains."‡

* See glossary.

† See glossary.

‡ i.e., no karmic record is kept. Only a master is a free man —one unbound by karma (the inexorable cosmic law that holds unenlightened persons accountable for their thoughts and actions). In urging Arjuna to fight on the battlefield, Lord Krishna assured him that he would incur no karma if he acted as God's agent, without egoistic consciousness.

A student found it difficult to conceive that God dwells within the flesh of man. The Master said:

"Just as coals, glowing red, reveal the presence of fire, so the marvelous mechanism of the body reveals the causative presence of Spirit."

· · ·

"Some persons think that unless a devotee undergoes great trials, he is not a saint. Others assert that a man of God-realization should be free from all suffering," the Master said during a lecture.

"The life of each master follows a certain unseen pattern. St. Francis was afflicted with diseases; the fully emancipated Christ allowed himself to be crucified. Other great personages, such as St. Thomas Aquinas and Lahiri Mahasaya,* passed their days without tremendous stress or tragedy.

"Saints attain final salvation from backgrounds vastly different. True sages demonstrate that, regardless of external conditions, they are able to reflect the Divine Image within them. They play whatever role God wills, whether or not it conforms to public opinion."

* See glossary.

A young hermitage resident loved to play pranks. Life to him was a continuous comedy. His merriment, welcome at times, occasionally prevented other devotees from serenely keeping their minds on God. One day Paramahansaji mildly scolded the boy.

"You should learn to be more serious," he remarked.

"Yes, Master," replied the disciple, sincerely regretting his restlessness. "But my habit is so strong! How can I change without your blessing?"

The Guru solemnly assured him:

"My blessing is there. God's blessing is there. Only your blessing is needed!"

.   .   .

"God understands you when everyone else misunderstands you," the Master said. "He is the Lover who cherishes you always, no matter what your mistakes. Others give you their affection for a while and then forsake you, but He abandons you never.

"In countless ways God is daily seeking your love. He doesn't punish you if you refuse Him, but you punish yourself. You find that 'all things betray thee, who betrayest Me.'"*

* *The Hound of Heaven,* by Francis Thompson.

"Sir, do you approve of church ceremonial?" a student inquired. The Master replied:

"Religious rites may help man to think of God, his Infinite Creator. But if there is too much ritual, everyone forgets what it is all about."

.   .   .

"What is God?" asked a student.

"God is Eternal Bliss," the Master replied. "His being is love, wisdom, and joy. He is both impersonal and personal, and manifests Himself in whatever way He pleases. He appears before His saints in the form each of them holds dear: a Christian sees Christ, a Hindu beholds Krishna* or the Divine Mother,* and so on. Devotees whose worship takes an impersonal turn become conscious of the Lord as an infinite Light or as the wondrous sound of *Aum*,* the primal Word, the Holy Ghost. The highest experience man can have is to feel that Bliss in which every other aspect of Divinity — love, wisdom, immortality — is fully contained.

"But how can I convey to you in words the nature of God? He is ineffable, indescribable. Only in deep meditation shall you know His unique essence."

* See glossary.

After a talk with an egotistical visitor, the Master remarked:

"The rains of God's mercy cannot gather on mountaintops of pride, but flow easily into valleys of humbleness."

•   •   •

Every time that the Master saw a certain disciple, who was decidedly the intellectual type, the Guru would say:

"Get devotion! Remember the words of Jesus: 'Father, thou hast hid these things from the wise and prudent, and hast revealed them unto babes.'"*

The disciple visited Master at his desert retreat shortly before Christmas of 1951. On a table lay some toys, intended for gifts. In a childlike spirit Paramahansaji played with them for a time, then asked the young man, "How do you like them?"

The disciple was still trying to get over his surprise; but he said, laughing, "They're fine, Sir." The Master smiled and quoted:

"'Suffer little children to come unto me, for of such is the kingdom of God.'"†

•   •   •

A student was dubious about his power of

* Matthew 11:25.   † Luke 18:16.

spiritual perseverance. To encourage him, Paramahansaji said:

"The Lord is not distant, but near. I see Him everywhere."

"But, Sir, you are a master!" the man protested.

"All souls are equal," the Guru replied. "The only difference between you and me is that I made the effort. I showed God that I love Him, and He came to me. Love is the magnet from which God cannot escape."

• • •

"Since you call your temple in Hollywood a 'church of all religions,' why do you place special emphasis on Christianity?" a visitor inquired.

"It is the wish of Babaji* that I do so," the Master said. "He asked me to interpret the Christian Bible and the Hindu Bible [Bhagavad-Gita], to point out the basic unity of the Christian and the Vedic† scriptures. He sent me to the West to fulfill that mission."

• • •

"A sin," the Master said, "is anything that keeps man oblivious of God."

* See glossary.
† See "Vedas" in glossary.

"Master, how could Jesus change water into wine?" a disciple asked. Sri Yogananda replied:

"The universe is the result of a play of light— vibrations of life energy. The motion pictures of creation, like scenes on a cinema screen, are projected and made visible through beams of light. Christ perceived the cosmical essence as light; in his eyes no essential difference existed between the light rays composing water and the light rays composing wine. Like God in the beginning of creation,* Jesus was able to command the vibrations of life energy to assume different forms.

"All men who overpass the delusory realms of relativity and duality enter the true world of Unity. They become one with Omnipotence, even as Christ said: 'He that believeth on me [he that knoweth the Christ Consciousness], the works that I do shall he do also: and greater works than these shall he do; because I go unto my Father [because I soon return to the Highest—the Vibrationless Absolute beyond creation, beyond phenomena].'"†

•   •   •

"Don't you believe in marriage, Master?" a student inquired. "You often talk as though you are against it." Paramahansaji replied:

---

* "Let there be light! And there was light."—Genesis 1:3.
† John 14:12. See "Sat-Tat-Aum" in glossary.

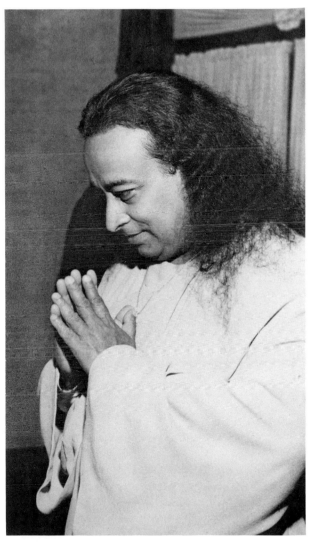

Paramahansa Yogananda at informal convocation of Self-Realization friends and members, Beverly Hills, California, 1949

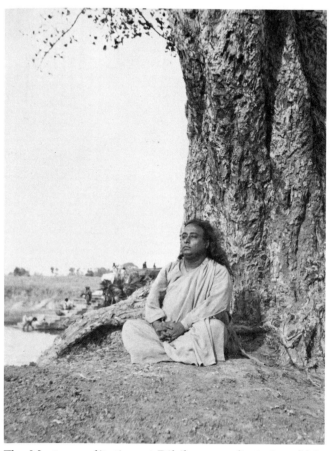

The Master meditating at Dihika, near first site of his school for boys, during visit to India, 1935. The school was relocated in Ranchi in 1918, where it continues to flourish.

"Marriage is unnecessary and hampering for those who, renunciants at heart, are intensely seeking God, the Eternal Lover. But in ordinary cases I am not against true marriage. Two persons who unite their lives to help each other toward divine realization are founding their marriage on the right basis: unconditional friendship. Woman is motivated primarily by feeling, and man by reason; marriage is meant to balance these qualities.

"Today there aren't many real soul unions, because young people get little spiritual training. Emotionally immature and unstable, they are usually influenced by fleeting sex attraction or worldly considerations that ignore the noble purpose of marriage." He added, "I often say: 'First establish yourself irrevocably on the divine path; then if you marry you won't make a mistake!'"

. . .

"Doesn't the Lord shower His grace more abundantly on certain men than on others?" a student inquired. Paramahansaji answered:

"God chooses those who choose Him."

. . .

Two ladies used to leave their automobile unlocked when they parked. The Master said to them, "Take proper precautions. Lock your car."

"Where is your faith in God?" they cried.

"I have faith," Paramahansaji answered. "It doesn't mean carelessness."

But they continued to leave the car unlocked. One day, when they had left many valuables on the back seat, thieves stole them.

"Why expect God to protect you if you ignore His laws of reason and caution?" the Master said. "Have faith, but be practical and don't tempt others."

• • •

Some of the disciples, caught up in a whirl of activity, were neglecting their meditation.* The Master cautioned them:

"Do not say: 'Tomorrow I will meditate longer.' You will suddenly find that a year has passed without fulfillment of your good intentions. Instead, say: 'This can wait and that can wait, but my search for God cannot wait.'"

• • •

"Sir," a disciple said, "how is it that some masters seem to know more than other masters?"

"All those who are fully liberated are equal in

* See "Kriya Yoga" in glossary.

wisdom," Paramahansaji replied. "They understand everything, but seldom reveal that knowledge. To please God they play the role He has assigned them. If they seem to blunder, it is because such conduct is part of their human role. Inwardly they are unaffected by the contrasts and relativities of *maya*."

•   •   •

"I find it difficult to keep the friendships I have made," a student confided.

"Choose your company carefully," Paramahansaji said. "Be cordial and sincere, but always maintain a little distance and reverence. Never be familiar with people. It is easy to make friends, but to keep friends you should follow this rule."

•   •   •

"Master," a student said, "can a soul be lost forever?" The Guru replied:

"That is impossible. Each soul is a part of God and is therefore imperishable."

•   •   •

"To a devotee on the right path, spiritual unfoldment is as natural and as unnoticed by him as his breathing," the Master said. "Once a man's heart is given to God, he becomes so deeply absorbed in Him that he scarcely realizes he has solved all of life's problems. Others begin to call him 'Guru.' In astonishment he thinks:

"'What! Has this sinner become a saint? Lord, may Thine image be so bright on my face that no one will see *me*, only *Thee!*'"

• • •

A certain student was given to constant self-examination for signs of spiritual progress. The Master said to him:

"If you plant a seed and dig it up daily to see if it is growing, it will never take root. Take proper care of it, but don't be curious!"

• • •

"What an odd person G——— is!" Several disciples were discussing the peculiarities of various persons. The Master said:

"Why be surprised? This world is just God's zoo."

• • •

"Aren't your teachings about controlling the emotions dangerous?" a student asked. "Many psychologists claim that suppression leads to mental maladjustments and even to physical illness."

The Master replied:

"Suppression is harmful — holding the thought that you want something but doing nothing constructive to get it. Self-control is beneficial — patiently replacing wrong thoughts by right ones, changing reprehensible actions to helpful ones.

"Those who dwell on evil hurt themselves. Men who fill their minds with wisdom and their lives with constructive activities spare themselves ignoble suffering."

．　．　．

"God tries us in all ways," the Master said. "He exposes our weaknesses, that we may become aware of them and transmute them into strengths. He may send us ordeals that appear insupportable; He may sometimes seem almost to be pushing us away. But the clever devotee will say:

"'No, Lord, I want Thee. Nothing shall deter me in my search. My heartfelt prayer is this: Never put me through the test of obliviousness of Thy presence.'"

"Sir, shall I ever leave the spiritual path?" inquired a doubt-filled disciple. The Master answered:

"How could you? Everyone in the world is on the spiritual path."

. . .

"Sir, give me the grace of devotion," a disciple asked pleadingly.

"In effect, you are saying: 'Give me money, so I can buy what I want,'" the Master replied. "But I say: 'No, first you have to *earn* the money. Then you may rightfully enjoy what you buy.'"

. . .

To help a discouraged student, the Master related this experience:

"One day I saw a big pile of sand on which a tiny ant was crawling. I said, 'The ant must be thinking it is scaling the Himalaya Mountains!' The pile may have seemed gigantic to the ant, but not to me. Similarly, a million of our solar years may be less than a minute in the mind of God. We should train ourselves to think in grand terms: Eternity! Infinity!"

Yoganandaji and a group of disciples were taking their evening exercise on the lawn of the Encinitas Hermitage. One of the young men inquired about a certain saint, whose name he did not know.

"Sir," he said, "it was the master who appeared before you here some months ago."

"I don't remember," Paramahansaji replied.

"It was out in the back garden, Sir."

"Many visit me there; I see some who have passed on, and some who are still on earth."

"How wonderful, Sir!"

"Wherever a devotee of God is, there His saints come." The Guru paused a minute or two while he did a few exercises. Then he said:

"Yesterday, while I was meditating in my room, I wanted to know certain things about the life of a great master of ancient times. He materialized before me. We sat on my bed for a long time, side by side, holding hands."

"Sir, did he tell you about his life?"

"Well," Paramahansaji answered, "in the interchange of vibration I got the whole picture."

• • •

To put renunciants of the Self-Realization Order* on their guard against spiritual complacency, the Master told them:

* See glossary.

"After one reaches *nirbikalpa samadhi** he never again falls into delusion. But until he attains that state he is not safe.

"A disciple of a famous Hindu master was such a great soul that his guru used to hold him up as an example for all to follow. One day the disciple mentioned that he was helping a devout woman by meditating with her.

"The Guru said quietly, 'Sadhu,* beware!'

"A few weeks later some seeds of bad karma* sprouted in the disciple's life; he ran away with the woman. He returned quickly to his guru, however, and cried, 'I am sorry!' He did not allow a mistake to become the center of his life, but put all errors behind him and redoubled his efforts for complete Self-realization.

"From this story you will see that it is possible for even a great devotee to sink temporarily into delusion. Never relax your vigilance until you are established in the Final Beatitude."

• • •

"Material science is more theoretical than true religion," the Master said. "Science is able to investigate, for example, the external nature and behavior of the atom. But the practice of meditation bestows omnipresence; a yogi can become one with the atom."

* See glossary.

A certain demanding disciple often arrived unexpectedly at the Mt. Washington Center,* and made frequent collect telephone calls to the Master. "He is a peculiar person," Paramahansaji once remarked. "But his heart is with the Lord. In spite of his faults he will reach his goal, because he won't let God alone until he does!"

* * *

When the Master first came to America he wore Indian dress, and his hair was long around his shoulders. Someone, fascinated by what was to him a strange sight, inquired, "Are you a fortune-teller?" Paramahansaji replied:

"No, I tell people how to mend their fortunes."

* * *

One day the Master told the disciples about a saint who fell from the highest path by public exhibition of miraculous powers. "He soon realized his mistake," Paramahansaji said, "and returned to his disciples. At the end of life he was a fully liberated soul."

"Sir, how did he rise again so quickly?" a devotee inquired. "Isn't the karmic punishment more severe for a man who falls from a state of

* Self-Realization Fellowship headquarters in Los Angeles, California. See glossary.

high advancement than for an ordinary person who acts wrongly in sheer ignorance? It seems strange that the Indian saint did not have to wait a long time for final liberation."

Smilingly the Master shook his head. "God is no tyrant," he said. "If a man was accustomed to a diet of ambrosia, he would be unhappy at having to eat stale cheese. If he cried brokenheartedly for ambrosia again, God wouldn't refuse him."

• • •

A friend thought it improper for Self-Realization Fellowship to advertise. The Master said:

"Wrigley uses ads to induce people to chew gum. Why shouldn't I use ads to induce people to 'chew' good ideas?"

• • •

Speaking of how quickly we may be released by God's grace from the delusions of *maya*, the Master said:

"In this world we seem to be immersed in a sea of troubles. Then the Divine Mother comes and shakes us, awakening us from this terrible dream. Every man, sooner or later, will have that liberating experience."

A student was wavering between the path of renunciation and a long-desired career. The Master said tenderly:

"All fulfillments you are seeking, and much more, are awaiting you in God."

•   •   •

To a student who appeared to be hopelessly enmeshed in bad habits, the Master suggested:

"If you lack will power, try to develop 'won't' power."

•   •   •

"What a responsibility one assumes when he tries to improve people!" exclaimed the Master. "The rose in the vase looks beautiful; one forgets all the gardening work that helped to make it beautiful. And if one must take pains in order to have a lovely rose, how much more effort is required to produce a perfect human being!"

•   •   •

"Don't mix with others too closely," the Master said. "Friendships do not satisfy us unless they are rooted in mutual love for the Lord.

"Our human wish for loving understanding from others is in reality the soul's desire for unity with God. The more we seek to satisfy that desire outwardly, the less likely we are to find the Divine Companion."

.   .   .

"There are three types of devotees," the Master said. "Believers who attend church and are satisfied; believers who live an upright life but make no effort to achieve oneness with God; and believers who are *determined* to discover their true identity."

.   .   .

Asked to define Self-realization, the Master said:

"Self-realization is the knowing — in body, mind, and soul—that we are one with the omnipresence of God; that we do not have to pray that it come to us, that we are not merely near it at all times, but that God's omnipresence is our omnipresence; that we are just as much a part of Him now as we ever will be. All we have to do is improve our knowing."

.   .   .

"God supplies quickly any need of His devotees, because they have eliminated the thwarting cross-currents of ego," the Master said.

"In the early days of the Mt. Washington Center, a mortgage payment was due; but we had no money in the bank. I prayed very deeply, telling the Lord: 'The welfare of the organization is in Thy hands.' The Divine Mother appeared before me. She said in English:

"'I am your stocks and bonds; I am your security.'

"A few days later I received in the mail a large donation for the Center."

·   ·   ·

One of the disciples was faithful and prompt in performing whatever tasks were given him by the Master; but for others he would do nothing. By way of correction, the Master said:

"You should serve others as you serve me. Remember, God dwells in all. Don't neglect any opportunity for pleasing Him."

·   ·   ·

"Death teaches us not to place our reliance on the flesh but on God. Therefore Death is a friend," the Master said. "We should not grieve unduly about the passing of our loved ones. It is selfish to desire that they always remain near us for our pleasure and comfort. Rather, rejoice that they have been summoned to advance toward soul freedom in the new and better environment of an astral world.*

"The sorrow of separation causes most men to cry for a while; then they forget. But the wise feel impelled to seek their vanished dear ones in the heart of the Eternal. What devotees lose in finite life, they find again in the Infinite."

• • •

"What is the best prayer?" a disciple inquired. The Master said:

"Say to the Lord: 'Please tell me Thy will.' Don't say: 'I want this and I want that,' but have faith that He knows what you need. You will see that you get much better things when He chooses for you."

• • •

The Master often asked the disciples to take charge of various minor matters. When one of them neglected such a little chore, thinking it unimportant, Paramahansaji gently chided her. He said:

"Faithfulness in the performance of small duties gives us strength to adhere to difficult determinations that life will someday force us to make."

* See glossary.

Paraphrasing a comment of Sri Yukteswar's,* the Master said to a new disciple:

"Some persons believe that entering a hermitage for self-discipline is as much cause for sorrow as a funeral. Instead, it may mean the funeral of all sorrow!"

• • •

"It is foolish to expect true happiness from earthly attachments and possessions, for they are powerless to bestow it," the Master said. "Yet millions of persons die of broken hearts, having tried vainly to find in worldly life the fulfillment that exists only in God, the Source of all joy."

• • •

Explaining why few men understand the Infinite God, the Master said:

"As a small cup cannot be a receptacle for the vast waters of an ocean, so the limited human mind cannot contain the universal Christ Consciousness. But when, by meditation, one continues to enlarge his mind, he finally attains omniscience. He becomes united with the Divine Intelligence that permeates the atoms of creation.

* *Autobiography of a Yogi,* Chapter 12.

"St. John said: 'As many as received him, to them gave he power to become the sons of God, even to them that believe on his name.'* St. John meant, by 'as many as received him,' those men who have perfected their power of receptivity to the Infinite; they alone regain their status as 'sons of God.' They 'believe on his name' by achieving oneness with Christ Consciousness."

•   •   •

A student who had once lived in the hermitage returned one day and said sadly to the Master:

"Why did I ever leave?"

"Isn't this a paradise, compared to the outside world?" Paramahansaji inquired.

"Indeed it is!" the young man replied, and sobbed so long that in sympathy the Master wept with him.

•   •   •

A sister of the Self-Realization Order complained of a lack of devotion. "It is not that I don't want to know God," she said, "but I seem unable to direct love toward Him. What should one do, who like myself is experiencing a 'dry' state?"

"You should not concentrate on the thought

* John 1:12.

that you lack devotion, but should work to develop it," the Master replied. "Why be upset because God hasn't shown Himself to you? Think of the long time you ignored Him!

"Meditate more; go deep; and follow the hermitage rules. By changing your habits you will awaken in your heart the memory of His wondrous Being; and, knowing Him, there is no doubt that you will love Him."

• • •

One Sunday the Master attended a church whose choir sang specially for him. After the services the choirmaster and the group asked Paramahansaji:

"Did you enjoy the singing?"

"It was all right," Sri Yogananda said, without enthusiasm.

"Oh! You didn't really like it?" they inquired.

"I wouldn't say that."

Pressed for an explanation, the Master finally said: "As far as technique was concerned, it was perfect; but you didn't realize to Whom you were singing. You were thinking only of pleasing me and the rest of the audience. The next time, sing not to man but to God."

With awe the disciples were discussing the sufferings gladly endured by the martyred saints of history. The Master said:

"The fate of the body is wholly unimportant to a man of God-realization. The physical form is like a plate that a devotee uses while he eats the wisdom-dinner of life. After his hunger has been eternally satisfied, of what worth is the plate? It may get broken, but the devotee hardly notices. He is absorbed in the Lord."

• • •

Long summer evenings often found the Master engaged in spiritual discussion with the disciples on the porch of the Encinitas Hermitage. On one such occasion the talk turned to miracles, and the Master said:

"Most men are interested in miracles and wish to see them. But my Master, Sri Yukteswarji, who had control over all natural forces, held very stern views on the subject. Just before I left India to lecture in America, he said to me: 'Arouse in men the love of God. Don't draw them to you by displays of unusual powers.'

"If I walked on fire and water, and filled every auditorium in the land with curiosity-seekers, what good would come of it? See the stars, the clouds, and the ocean; see the mist on the grass. Can any miracle of man compare with these essentially inexplicable phenomena? Even so, few men are led through nature to love God—the Miracle of all miracles."

•   •   •

To a group of rather procrastinating young disciples, the Master said:

"You should methodize your life. God created routine. The sun shines till dusk and the stars shine till dawn."

•   •   •

"Isn't the wisdom of saints due to their receiving the Lord's special favor?" a visitor inquired.

"No," the Master replied. "That some persons have less divine realization than others is not because God limits the flow of His grace, but because most men prevent His ever-present light from passing freely through them. By removing the dark screen of egotism, all His children may equally reflect His rays of omniscience."

•   •   •

A visitor spoke disparagingly of India's so-called idol worship. The Master quietly said:

"If a man, sitting with closed eyes in a church, allows his thoughts to dwell on worldly matters—

the idols of materialism—God is aware that He is not being worshiped.

"If a man, bowing before a stone image, sees it as a symbol and reminder of the living omnipresent Spirit, God accepts that worship."

. . .

"I am going to the hills to be alone with God," a student informed the Master.

"You will not advance spiritually in that way," Paramahansaji replied. "Your mind is not yet ready to concentrate deeply on Spirit. Your thoughts will dwell mostly on memories of people and worldly pastimes, even though you remain in a cave. Cheerful performance of your earthly duties, coupled with daily meditation, is the better path."

. . .

After praising a disciple, the Master said:

"When you are told you are good, you should not relax but should try to become even better. Your continuous improvement gives happiness to you, to those around you, and to God."

. . .

"Renunciation is not negative but positive. It

isn't the giving up of anything except misery," the Master said.

"One should not think of renunciation as a path of sacrifice. Rather it is a divine investment, by which our few cents of self-discipline will yield a million spiritual dollars. Is it not wisdom to spend the gold coins of our fleeting days to purchase Eternity?"

· · ·

Gazing one Sunday morning at the masses of blossoms that decorated the temple, the Master said:

"Because God is Beauty, He created loveliness in the flowers that they might speak of Him. More than anything else in nature they hint at His presence. His shining face peeks out of the windows of lilies and forget-me-nots. In the fragrance of the rose He seems to say: 'Seek Me.' That is His mode of speech; otherwise He remains silent. He shows His handiwork in the beauty of creation, but doesn't reveal that He Himself is hidden there."

· · ·

Two hermitage disciples asked the Master's permission to take a trip to visit friends. Paramahansaji replied:

"In the beginning of a renunciant's training, it is not good for him to mix often with worldly people. His mind becomes leaky, like a sieve, and cannot hold the waters of God-perception. Taking trips will not bring you realization of the Infinite."

Because it was the Guru's way to give suggestions, not commands, he added, "It is my duty to warn you when I see that you are turning in the wrong direction. But do what you will."

• • •

"On earth God is trying to evolve the universal art of right living by encouraging in men's hearts feelings of brotherhood and appreciation for others," the Master said. "He has therefore permitted no nation to be complete in itself. To the members of each race He has given some special aptitude, some unique genius, with which they may make a distinctive contribution to the world civilization.

"Peace on earth will be hastened by a constructive exchange among nations of their best features. Ignoring the faults of a race, we should discern and emulate its virtues. It is important to note that the great saints of history have personified the ideals of all lands, and have embodied the highest aspirations of all religions."

• • •

The Master's conversation sparkled with similes. One day he said:

"I see those on the spiritual path as though in a race. Some are sprinting; others are moving along slowly. A number are even running backward!"

Another time he remarked:

"Life is a battle. Men are fighting their inward enemies of greed and ignorance. Many are wounded — with bullets of desires."

• • •

Paramahansaji had chastised several disciples for a lack of efficiency in the performance of their duties. They were feeling very sad; and then the Guru said:

"I do not like to scold you, for all of you are so good. But when I see specks on a white wall I want to remove them."

• • •

Paramahansaji and a few others were traveling by auto to visit a Self-Realization retreat. An old man, pack on back, was trudging along the hot, dusty road. The Master asked that the car be stopped, called the man, and gave him some money. A few minutes later Paramahansaji said to the disciples:

"The world and its terrible surprises! We ride while such an old man walks. All of you should resolve to escape from fear of the unpredictable turns of *maya*. If that unfortunate fellow had God-realization, poverty or riches would not matter. In the Infinite all states of consciousness are transmuted into one: Ever New Bliss."

• • •

"Sir, what passage in *Autobiography of a Yogi* do you consider the most inspiring for the average man?" a student asked. The Master reflected for a while, then said:

"These words of my guru, Sri Yukteswar: 'Forget the past. Human conduct is ever unreliable until man is anchored in the Divine. Everything in future will improve if you are making a spiritual effort now.'"

• • •

"God remembers us, though we remember Him not," the Master said. "If He forgot creation for a second, everything would disappear tracelessly. Who but He holds in the sky this mud ball of earth? Who but He impels the growth of trees and flowers? It is the Lord alone who maintains the beat of our hearts, digests our food, and daily renews our body cells. Yet how few of His children give Him a thought!"

"The mind," Paramahansaji said, "is like a miraculous rubber band that can be expanded to infinity without breaking."

.   .   .

"How can a saint take on himself the bad karma* of others?" a student asked. The Master replied:

"If you saw that a man was going to hit another, you could step in front of the intended victim and let the blow fall on you. That is what a great master does. He perceives, in the lives of his devotees, when unfavorable effects of their past bad karma are about to descend on them. If he thinks it wise, he employs a certain metaphysical method by which he transfers to himself the consequences of his disciples' errors. The law of cause and effect operates mechanically or mathematically; yogis understand how to switch its currents.

"Because saints are conscious of God as Eternal Being and Inexhaustible Life Energy, they are able to survive blows that would kill an ordinary man. Their minds are unaffected by physical disease or worldly misfortunes."

* See glossary. The law of transfer of karma is explained more fully in Chapter 21 of *Autobiography of a Yogi*.

The Master was discussing with disciples plans for expansion of the Self-Realization Fellowship work. He said:

"Remember, the church is the hive, but the Lord is the Honey. Do not be satisfied with telling people about spiritual truths; show them how they themselves may attain God-consciousness."

• • •

Paramahansaji was nonattached, yet loving and ever faithful. One day he said:

"When I don't see my friends I don't miss them; but when I see them I never tire of them."

• • •

"I see the Lord in His universe," the Master said. "Viewing a beautiful tree, my heart is moved and whispers: 'He is there!' I bow to adore Him. Doesn't He permeate every atom of the earth? Could our planet exist at all except by the cohesive power of God? A true devotee sees Him in all persons, in all things; each rock becomes an altar.

"When the Lord commanded: 'Thou shalt have no other gods before me. Thou shalt not make unto thee any graven image,'* He meant that we should not exalt the objects of creation above

* Exodus 20:3–4.

the Creator. Our love for Nature, family, friends, duties, and possessions should not occupy the supreme throne in our hearts. That is where *God* belongs."

• • •

After pointing out a disciple's error, the Master said:

"You should not feel sensitive about my correcting you. It is because you are winning in the battle against ego-guided habits that I continue to show you the way of self-discipline. I bless you continually for a glorious future in good. I have cautioned you this evening, lest you get used to mechanical performance of your spiritual duties and forget to make daily a deep, ardent effort to find God."

• • •

A minister from another church called on Paramahansaji one evening. The visitor said dejectedly:

"I am so confused in my spiritual thinking!"

"Then why do you preach?"

"I like preaching."

"Didn't Christ tell us that the blind should not lead the blind?"* the Master said. "Your

---

* Matthew 15:14.

doubts will vanish if you learn and practice the method of meditation on God, the Sole Certainty. Without inspiration from Him, how can you convey divine realizations to others?"

●　　●　　●

The disciples were listening eagerly, in the main hall of the Encinitas Hermitage, as the Master talked far into the night on sublime subjects.

"I am here to tell you of the joy to be found in God," he concluded, "the joy that each of you is free to discover, the joy that permeates me every moment of my life. For He walks with me, He talks with me, He thinks with me, He plays with me, He guides me in all ways. 'Lord,' I say to Him, 'I have no troubles; Thou art ever with me. I am happy to be Thy servant, a humble instrument to help Thy children. Whatever persons or happenings Thou dost bring to me are Thy responsibility; I will not interfere with Thy plan for me by harboring desires of my own.' "

●　　●　　●

"I know, deep within me, that I'll find happiness only in God. Yet many earthly things still attract me," said a young man who was contemplating entering the Self-Realization Order.

"A child thinks it's fun to play with mud pies, but loses interest in them when he is older," the

Master replied. "When you grow up spiritually you won't miss the pleasures of the world."

• • •

After a visit with several learned men, the Master said to the disciples:

"A number of intellectuals who quote the prophets are like victrolas. Just as a machine plays records of sacred writings without understanding their meaning, so many scholars who repeat Holy Writ are unaware of its true significance. They do not see the deep, life-transforming values of the scriptures. From their reading such men gain, not God-realization, but only a knowledge of *words*. They become proud and argumentative."

He added, "That is why I tell all of you to read less and to meditate more."

• • •

The Master said: "In creation it appears that God sleeps in the minerals, dreams in the flowers, awakens in the animals, and in man* *knows* that He is awake."

---

* "The human body was not solely a result of evolution from beasts, but was produced through an act of special creation by God. The animal forms were too crude to express full divinity; man was uniquely given acutely awakened occult centers in the spine, and the potentially omniscient 'thousand-petaled lotus' in the brain."—*Autobiography of a Yogi.*

The Master had given unstintingly of his time
to disciples and truth seekers. Then he sought the
solitary peace of a Self-Realization retreat in the
desert. When he and a small group reached their
destination, and the car motor had been turned
off, Paramahansaji remained quietly in the auto.
He seemed to be immersing himself in the vast
silence of night in the desert. Finally he said:

"Wherever there is a well, thirsty people
gather. But sometimes, for a change, the well likes
to be unfrequented."

* * *

"Within your physical form is a secret door to
divinity,"* the Master said. "Hasten your evolution by proper diet, healthful living, and reverence for your body as a temple of God. Unlock its
sacred spinal door by the practice of scientific
meditation."

* The Lord has equipped the body of man, alone among His
creatures, with secret spinal centers whose awakening (by
yoga or, in some cases, by intense devotional fervor) confers
divine illumination. The Hindu scriptures therefore teach
(1) that a human body is a precious gift, and (2) that man
cannot work out his material karma except in physical
encasement. He will reincarnate on this earth again and
again, until he is a master. Only then shall the human body
have fulfilled the purpose for which it was created. (See
"reincarnation" in glossary.)

"I have always desired to seek God, Master, but I want to get married," a student said. "Don't you think I can still attain the Divine Goal?"

"A young person who prefers to have a family first, thinking he will seek God afterward, may be making a grave error," the Master replied. "In ancient India children were given instruction in self-discipline in a hermitage. Today, all over the world, such training is lacking. The modern man has little control over his senses, impulses, moods, and desires. He is quickly influenced by his environment. In the natural course of events he enters the householder's state and becomes overburdened with worldly duties. He usually forgets to say even a tiny prayer to God."

• • •

"Why is suffering so widespread on earth?" a student asked. The Master replied:

"There are many reasons for suffering. One reason is to prevent man from learning too much of others and not enough of himself. Pain eventually compels human beings to wonder: 'Is a cause-effect principle operating in my life? Are my troubles due to my wrong thinking?'"

• • •

Realizing the burden a saint assumes to aid others, a student said one day to Paramahansaji:

"Sir, when the time comes, undoubtedly you

will be glad to leave this earth and never return."

"So long as people in this world are crying for help, I shall return to ply my boat and offer to take them to the heavenly shores," the Guru replied.

"Should I glory in freedom while others are suffering? Knowing that they are in misery (even as I myself would be had God not shown me His grace), I could not fully enjoy even His ineffable beatitude."

• • •

"Avoid a negative approach to life," the Master told a group of disciples. "Why gaze down the sewers when there is loveliness all around us? One may find some fault in even the greatest masterpieces of art, music, and literature. But isn't it better to enjoy their charm and glory?

"Life has a bright side and a dark side, for the world of relativity is composed of light and shadows. If you permit your thoughts to dwell on evil, you yourself will become ugly. Look only for the good in everything, that you absorb the quality of beauty."

• • •

"Master, I am conscious only of the present life. Why have I no recollection of previous incarnations* and no foreknowledge of a future exis-

* See "reincarnation" in glossary.

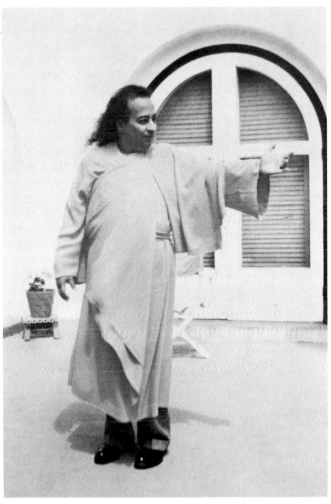

Paramahansaji gestures a warm greeting to members outside
Self-Realization Temple, San Diego, California, 1949

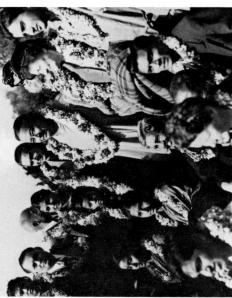

Paramahansaji with guests Amala and Uday Shankar, distinguished Hindu classical dance artists, and their company of dancers and musicians (the brilliant sitarist Ravi Shankar is at lower left); Self-Realization Ashram Center, Encinitas, California, 1950

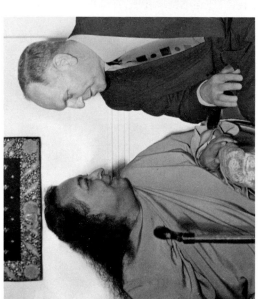

Sri Yogananda and former California Lt. Governor Goodwin J. Knight, who took part in dedication of India Hall at Hollywood Self-Realization Ashram Center, 1951

tence?" a disciple inquired. Paramahansaji replied:

"Life is like a great chain in the ocean of God. When a portion of the chain is pulled out of the waters you see only that small part. The beginning and the end are hidden. In this incarnation you are viewing only one link in the chain of life. The past and the future, though invisible, remain in the deeps of God. He reveals their secrets to devotees who are in tune with Him."

•　•　•

"Do you believe in the divinity of Christ?" a visitor inquired. The Master replied:

"Yes. I love to talk of him because he was a man of perfect Self-realization. However, he was not the *only* son of God, nor did he claim to be. Instead, he clearly taught that those who do the will of God become, like himself, one with Him. Wasn't it the mission of Jesus on earth to remind all men that the Lord is their Heavenly Father, and to show them the way back to Him?"

•　•　•

"It does not seem right that the Heavenly Father should allow so much misery in the world," a student remarked. Paramahansaji replied:

"No cruelty exists in God's plan, because in

His eyes there is no good or evil—only pictures of light and shadows. The Lord intended us to view the dualistic scenes of life as He does Himself—the ever joyous Witness of a stupendous cosmic drama.

"Man has falsely identified himself with the pseudo-soul or ego. When he transfers his sense of identity to his true being, the immortal soul, he discovers that all pain is unreal. He no longer can even *imagine* the state of suffering."

The Guru added: "Great masters who come to earth to help their bewildered brothers are permitted by God to share, on a certain level of their minds, the sorrows of mankind; but that sympathetic participation in human feelings does not disturb deeper levels of consciousness on which saints experience only changeless beatitude."

· · ·

To devotees the Master often said: "A song you should constantly hum, unheard by any, is: 'My Lord, I will be Thine always.'"

· · ·

A devotee had decided to leave the hermitage. He said to Paramahansaji:

"No matter where I am, I will always meditate and follow your teachings."

"No, you won't be able to do it," the Master answered. "Your place is here. If you return to your old life, you will forget this path."

The student departed. He failed to continue the practice of meditation and immersed himself in worldliness. The Guru grieved about his "lost sheep." To the disciples he said:

"Evil has its power. If you side with it, it will hold you. When you make a misstep, return immediately to the ways of righteousness."

•　•　•

"If a man told you: 'I am God,' you would not feel he was speaking the truth," the Master said to a group of disciples. "But we all may rightly say: 'God has become me.' Of what other substance could we be made? He is the sole fabric of creation. Before He brought into manifestation the phenomenal worlds, nothing existed except Himself as Spirit. From His being He created all: the universe and the souls of men."

•　•　•

"Should I read books?" a disciple asked.

"Scriptural study will inspire in you a greater zeal for God, if you read the stanzas slowly and try to assimilate their deep meaning," the Master replied. "Reading sacred literature without following its precepts produces vanity, false satisfaction, and what I call 'intellectual indigestion.'

"Many persons are required to give their attention to secular books, in order to make a living; but renunciants like yourself should not read undevotional writings, those without God in their pages."

•   •   •

"Does creation really go through a process of evolution?" a disciple asked.

"Evolution is a suggestion of God in the human mind, and is true in the world of relativity," the Master replied. "Actually, everything is taking place in the present. In Spirit there is no evolution, just as there is no change in the beam of light through which all the developing scenes of cinema pictures are manifested. The Lord can turn the motion picture of creation backward or forward, but everything is really happening in an eternal *now*."

•   •   •

"Does working for the Lord and not for self mean that it's wrong to be ambitious?" inquired a disciple.

"No, you should be ambitious to accomplish work for God," the Master said. "If your will is weak and your ambition dead, you have lost life already. But don't let ambition produce worldly attachment.

"To seek things only for yourself is destructive; to seek things for others is expansive; but to seek to please God is the best attitude. It will lead you directly into the Divine Presence."

•   •   •

"I am attracted to hermitage life," a man said to Paramahansaji, "but I hesitate to give up my freedom."

"Without God-realization you have little freedom," the Master replied. "Your life is ruled by impulse, whims, moods, habits, and environment. By following the advice of a guru, and by accepting his discipline, you will gradually emerge from sense slavery. Freedom means the power to act by soul guidance, not by the compulsions of desires and habits. Obeying the ego leads to bondage; obeying the soul brings liberation."

•   •   •

"Sir, is there a scientific method, apart from *Kriya Yoga*, that will lead a devotee to God?" a student inquired.

"Yes," the Master said. "A sure and swift way to the Infinite is to keep one's attention at the Christ Consciousness* center between the eyebrows."

* See "spiritual eye" in glossary.

"Is it wrong to doubt? I don't like to believe blindly," a student said. The Master replied:

"There are two kinds of doubt: destructive and constructive. Destructive doubt is habitual skepticism. Men who cultivate that attitude disbelieve blindly; they shun the work of impartial investigation. Skepticism is a static on one's mental radio that causes him to lose the program of truth.

"Constructive doubt is intelligent questioning and fair examination. Those who cultivate that attitude do not prejudge matters or accept as valid the opinions of others. In the spiritual path, constructive doubters base their conclusions on tests and personal experience: the proper approach to truth."

. . .

"Why should God surrender Himself easily to you?" the Master said during a lecture. "You who work so hard for money and so little for divine realization! The Hindu saints tell us that if we would give so short a time as twenty-four hours to continuous, uninterrupted prayer, the Lord would appear before us or make Himself known to us in some other way. If we devote even one hour daily to deep meditation on Him, in time He will come to us."

Paramahansaji had advised a certain disciple, intellectually inclined, to try to develop devotion. Feeling that the young man was making good progress, one day the Master said to him lovingly:

"Keep steadily on the devotional path. How 'dry' your life was when you depended only on intellect!"

. . .

"Desires are the most unrelenting enemies of man; he cannot appease them," the Master said. "Have only one desire: to know God. Satisfying the sensory desires cannot satisfy you, because you are not the senses. They are only your servants, not your Self."

. . .

As Paramahansaji and the disciples sat near the fireplace in the hermitage drawing room, talking on spiritual subjects, the Master said:

"Picture two men. On their right is the valley of life, and on their left is the valley of death. Both are men of reason, but one goes right and the other goes left. Why? Because one has used correctly his power of discrimination, and the other has misused that power by indulging in false rationalizations."

"Master, Dr. Lewis was your first disciple in this country, wasn't he?"

Paramahansaji answered, "That's what they say." Seeing that the questioner was a little taken aback, the Master added, "I never say that others are my disciples. God is the Guru; they are His disciples."

•   •   •

A student deplored the fact that reports of the evil in the world were usually predominant in the newspapers.

"Evil spreads with the wind," the Master said. "Truth is able to travel against the wind."

•   •   •

Many persons were curious to know the Master's age. He would laugh and say:

"I have no age. I existed before the atoms, before the dawn of creation."

To the disciples he gave this counsel:

"Tell yourselves this truth: 'I am the infinite Ocean, become many in the waves. I am eternal and immortal. I am Spirit.'"

"What keeps the earth from leaving its orbit?" Paramahansaji asked a disciple.

"The centripetal force or gravitational attraction of the sun, Sir, which prevents the earth from being lost in outer space," the young man answered.

"What, then, keeps the earth from being fully drawn into the sun?" the Master went on.

"The centrifugal force in the earth, Sir, by which it maintains a certain distance from the sun."

The Master smiled significantly. Later the devotee realized that Paramahansaji had been speaking in allegory of God as the attractive Sun, and egoistic man as the earth that "maintains distance."

•   •   •

A student was trying to grasp by mental analysis what God is. The Master said:

"Do not think that you can comprehend the Infinite Lord by reason. Reason can grasp only the cause-effect principle that pertains to the phenomenal worlds. Reason is powerless to understand transcendental truth and the nature of the Causeless Absolute.

"Man's highest faculty is not reason but intuition: apprehension of knowledge derived immediately and spontaneously from the soul, not from the fallible agency of the senses or of reason."

•   •   •

Settling a dispute between two students, the Master said, "Mankind has only one real enemy—ignorance. Let us all work together for its destruction, helping and cheering one another along the way."

•   •   •

"How could God, the Unmanifested Absolute, appear in visible form* to a devotee?" a man asked. The Master said:

"If you doubt, you won't see; and if you see, you won't doubt."

•   •   •

"But, Sir," pleaded a disciple, "I didn't realize that my words would cause M——— unhappiness." The Master replied:

"Even though we unknowingly break a law or unintentionally hurt someone, we have nevertheless given offense. It is egotism that misdirects us. Saints do not act unwisely, because they have forsaken the ego and have found their true identity in God."

* See "Divine Mother" in glossary.

A disciple expressed disgust for a person whose crimes had been recently discussed in the newspapers.

"I am sorry for a man who is sick," the Master said. "Why should I hate a man who has fallen into evil? He is *really* sick."

• • •

"When the walls of a reservoir are destroyed," the Master said, "the waters rush out in all directions. Similarly, when the limitations of restlessness* and delusion are removed by meditation, the consciousness of man spreads out to infinity and merges in the omnipresence of Spirit."

• • •

"Why does the Lord give us families if He doesn't want us to love them more than we love other persons?" a student asked.

"By placing us in families, God affords us an opportunity to overcome selfishness and to find it easier to think of others," the Master replied. "In friendships He offers us a way to broaden further our sympathies. Even that is not the end; we should continue to expand our love until it becomes divine, encompassing all beings everywhere. Otherwise, how may we achieve oneness with God, the Father of all?"

* See "breath" in glossary.

God's patient love found poignant expression when the Guru said: "In one of His aspects, a very touching aspect, the Lord may be said to be a beggar. He yearns for our attention. The Master of the Universe, at whose glance all stars, suns, moons, and planets quiver, is running after man and saying: 'Won't you give Me your affection? Don't you love Me, the Giver, more than the things I have made for you? Won't you seek Me?'

"But man says: 'I am too busy now; I have work to do. I can't take time to look for You.'

"And the Lord says: 'I will wait.'"

.   .   .

The Master gave a talk about creation and why the Lord had started it. The disciples asked many questions. Paramahansaji laughed and said:

"This life is a master novel, written by God, and man would go crazy if he tried to understand it by reason alone. That is why I tell you to meditate more. Enlarge the magic cup of your intuition and then you will be able to hold the ocean of infinite wisdom."

.   .   .

"I understand you have two kinds of members—those who live in the world, and renunciants who live in the hermitage," said a visitor. "Which kind is following the better way?"

"Some persons love God so deeply that nothing else matters. They become renunciants and work here for the Lord only," the Master replied. "Those who must work in the world to support themselves and their families are not debarred from divine communion. Ordinarily it will take them longer to find God, that's all."

* * *

A man lamented that things were going badly for him. "It must be my karma," he said. "I can't seem to succeed in anything."

"Then you should make a greater effort," the Master replied. "Forget the past, and trust more in God. Our fate is not predestined by Him; nor is karma the sole factor, though our lives are *influenced* by our past thoughts and past activities. If you are not happy with the way life is turning out, change the pattern. I don't like to hear men sigh and ascribe present failure to past-life errors; to do so is spiritual laziness. Get busy and weed the garden of your life."

* * *

"Why doesn't God punish those who blaspheme His name?" a student inquired. The Master said:

"God is moved neither by insincere prayers and praise nor by ignorant atheistical outbursts. He answers man only through law. Hit a stone with your knuckles, drink sulphuric acid, and you must bear the consequences. Break His laws of life, and suffering will come. Think rightly, behave nobly, and peace will come. Love God unconditionally and *He* will come!"

· · ·

"The greatest man is he who considers himself to be the least, as Jesus taught," Paramahansaji said. "A real leader is one who first learned obedience to others, who feels himself to be the servant of all, and who never puts himself on a pedestal. Those who want flattery don't deserve our admiration, but he who serves us has a right to our love. Isn't God the servant of His children, and does He ask for praise? No, He is too great to be moved by it."

· · ·

The Master was giving advice to Self-Realization ministers about preparing their sermons. He said:

"First, meditate deeply. Then, holding to the feeling of peace that comes with meditation, think about the subject of your talk. Write down your ideas and include one or two funny stories, because people like to laugh; and finish with a quotation from the *SRF Lessons*.* Then put your notes away and forget the matter. Just before you give your sermon in the church, ask the Spirit to flow through your words. In these ways you will draw inspiration not from the ego but from God."

. . .

A woman told the Guru that, although she attended his temple services regularly, she did not feel closer to God. Paramahansaji replied:

"If I tell you that a fruit has a certain color, and that it is sweet, and how it grows, you still understand only the nonessentials about it. To know its distinctive flavor you yourself must eat it. Similarly, to realize truth you must experience it."

He added: "I can only arouse your appetite for divine fruit. Why don't you get busy and take a bite?"

. . .

"We are all waves on the bosom of the Ocean," the Master said. "The sea can exist without the waves, but the waves cannot exist without the sea. Similarly, Spirit can exist without man, but man cannot exist without Spirit."

* See glossary.

A devotee was struggling, without much success, to overcome his weaknesses. To him the Master said:

"At present I don't ask you to overcome *maya*. All I ask is that you *resist* it."

• • •

To a new student, eager to escape the trials of life, the Master said:

"The Divine Physician is keeping you in the hospital of earthly delusion until your disease of desire for material things is cured. Then He will let you go Home."

• • •

During a lecture on the east coast, the Master met a prominent businessman. In the course of their conversation, the man remarked:

"I am disgustingly healthy and disgustingly wealthy."

"But you are not disgustingly happy, are you?" the Master responded.

The man conceded the point and became a devoted student of Paramahansaji's *Kriya Yoga* teachings.

• • •

Referring to the Biblical passage, "Behold, I stand at the door, and knock: if any man hear my voice, and open the door, I will come in to him, and will sup with him, and he with me,"* the Master said:

"Christ is seeking to enter the door of your heart, but you have latched it with indifference."

.   .   .

"It is good, Sir, that you are preaching in America at this time. After two world wars, people are more receptive to your spiritual message," remarked a man who had recently read *Autobiography of a Yogi*.

"Yes," the Master replied. "Fifty years ago they would have been indifferent. 'To every thing there is a season, and a time to every purpose under the heaven.'"†

.   .   .

With the rapid growth of Self-Realization Fellowship, the organization he had founded to disseminate his teachings, the Master observed that some of the disciples were becoming engrossed in work. He cautioned them, "Never be too busy to sing secretly to the Lord: 'Thou art mine; I am Thine.'"

* Revelation 3:20.
† Ecclesiastes 3:1.

Observing that a disciple had lapsed into a sad mood, the Master said gently:

"When the thorn of misery is piercing your heart, take it out with the thorn of meditation."

• • •

"This is not a path for the idle," the Master said, during a little speech of welcome to a new resident at the Mt. Washington Center. "The indolent cannot find God, the Prodigious Laborer in creation! He doesn't help those who think He should do all the work. He secretly aids those who perform their duties cheerfully and intelligently, and who say: 'Lord, it is Thou who art using my brain and hands.'"

• • •

A student complained that he was too busy to meditate. The Master's reply was succinct:

"Suppose God were too busy to look after you?"

• • •

"The human body is a divine idea in the mind of God," the Master said. "He made us from rays of immortal light* and encased us in a bulb of flesh. We have placed our attention on the

---

* "If therefore thine eye be single, *thy whole body shall be full of light.*" — Matthew 6:22.

frailties of the perishable bulb rather than on the eternal life energy within it."

• • •

"God seems vague and far away," a student argued.

"The Lord seems distant only because your attention is directed outward to His creation and not inward to Him," the Master said. "Whenever your mind wanders in the maze of myriad worldly thoughts, patiently lead it back to remembrance of the indwelling Lord. In time you will find Him ever with you — a God who talks with you in your own language, a God whose face peeps at you from every flower and shrub and blade of grass.

"Then you shall say: 'I am free! I am clothed in the gossamer of Spirit; I fly from earth to heaven on wings of light.' And what joy will consume your being!"

• • •

"Can you tell just by looking at a person how far he has advanced spiritually?" a disciple asked Paramahansaji.

"At once," the Master quietly replied. "I see the hidden side of people, because that's my work in life. But I don't talk about my findings. He who egotistically says he knows, knows not. He who really knows, because he knows God, remains silent."

•   •   •

To a disciple who repeatedly asked the Master to give her God-consciousness, yet did nothing to prepare herself for such a state, the Master said:

"A true lover of God can inspire his truant brothers and sisters with a desire to return to their home in Him; but they themselves, step by step, must make the actual journey."

•   •   •

Every year, on the day before Christmas, the disciples would gather with the Master at the Mount Washington Center for meditation. The sacred session usually lasted all day and into the evening hours. During the Christmas meditation in 1948 the Divine Mother appeared to the Master, and the awed disciples heard him speaking to Her. Many times he exclaimed, with a deep sigh:

"Oh, You are so beautiful!"

Paramahansaji told many of the devotees present Her wishes concerning their lives. Suddenly he cried:

"Don't go! You say the subconscious material

desires of these people are driving You away? Oh, come back! Come back!"

• • •

"I have never been able to believe in heaven, Master," a new student remarked. "Is there truly such a place?"

"Yes," Paramahansaji replied. "Those who love God and put their trust in Him go there when they die. On that astral plane,* one has power to materialize anything immediately by sheer thought. The astral body is made of shimmering light. In those realms colors and sounds exist that earth knows nothing about. It is a beautiful and enjoyable world, but even the experience of heaven is not the highest state. Man attains final beatitude when he overpasses the phenomenal spheres and realizes God, and himself, as Absolute Spirit."

• • •

"The diamond and the charcoal lying side by side equally receive the sun's rays; but until the charcoal becomes a diamond, white and clear, it cannot reflect the sunlight," the Master said. "Similarly, the ordinary person, spiritually dark, cannot be compared in beauty with the purified devotee who is able to reflect the light of God."

* See "astral worlds" in glossary.

"Refrain from gossip and the spreading of rumors," the Master told a group of disciples. "Give a lie a twenty-four-hour start and sometimes it seems to become immortal.

"A man who once lived in the hermitage often told untruths about others. One day he started a baseless rumor about a boy. When it reached my ears, I whispered to a few persons a harmless but false story about the man.

"He came to me and said indignantly: 'Listen to what all the people here are saying about me!' I listened politely. When he was through I remarked:

"'You don't like it, do you?'

"'Of course not!'

"'Now you know how the boy felt when others were repeating the lie you had told about him.' The man was abashed. I went on, 'It was I who first put in circulation that story about you. I did it to teach you a lesson in consideration for others—a lesson that you have been unable to learn in any other way.'"

•   •   •

"You should go deep in meditation," the Master said to a group of disciples. "As soon as you allow yourself to become restless, the old troubles start again: desires for sex, wine, and money."

"Man seems to have little free will," a student observed. "My life is 'set' in so many ways."

"Turn toward God and you will find yourself shaking off the chains of habits and environment," the Master replied. "Though the drama of life is governed by a cosmic plan, man may change his part by changing his center of consciousness. The Self identified with the ego is bound; the Self identified with the soul is free."

. . .

A visitor to the Mt. Washington Center said to Paramahansaji:

"I believe in God. But He doesn't help me."

"Belief in God and faith in God are different," the Master replied. "A belief is valueless if you don't test it and live by it. Belief converted into experience becomes faith. That is why the prophet Malachi told us: *'Prove me now herewith,* saith the Lord of hosts, if I will not open you the windows of heaven, and pour you out a blessing, that there shall not be room enough to receive it.'"*

. . .

A student had made a serious error. She lamented, "I have always cultivated good habits. It

* Malachi 3:10.

seems incredible that this misfortune should have happened to me."

"Your mistake was to rely too heavily on good habits and to neglect constant exercise of right judgment," the Master said. "Your good habits help you in ordinary and familiar situations but may not suffice to guide you when a new problem arises. Then discrimination is necessary. By deeper meditation you will learn to choose the right course in everything, even when confronted by extraordinary circumstances." He added:

"Man is not an automaton, and therefore cannot always live wisely by simply following set rules and rigid moral precepts. In the great variety of daily problems and events, we find scope for the development of good judgment."

• • •

One day Paramahansaji censured a monk for misbehavior. The disciple asked, "But you will forgive me, won't you, Sir?"

The Master said, "Well, what else can I do?"

• • •

A large group of women disciples, old and young, were enjoying a picnic with the Master on the grounds of the Self-Realization Ashram Center in Encinitas, overlooking the Pacific Ocean. Paramahansaji said:

"How much better this is than the time-wasting amusements of restless worldly people. Each of you is becoming rich in peace and happiness. God wants His children to live simply and to be content with innocent pleasures."

• • •

"Don't concern yourself with the faults of others," the Master said. "Use the scouring powder of wisdom to keep the rooms of your own mind bright and spotless. By your example, other persons will be inspired to do their own house-cleaning."

• • •

Two disciples, unjustly angry with one of their brothers, took their complaints to the Master. He listened in silence. When they were through, he said, "Change yourselves."

• • •

"Train the will of your children in the right direction, away from selfishness and consequent unhappiness," the Master said to a mother. "Don't curtail their freedom or oppose them unnecessarily. Give them your suggestions with love and with understanding of the importance to them of their own little desires. If you chastise them instead of reasoning with them, you will lose their confidence. If a child is stubborn, explain your viewpoint to him once and then say nothing more. Let him get his own little hard knocks; they will teach him discrimination quicker than would any words of counsel."

[In training his spiritual family of disciples, Paramahansaji followed his own advice. He helped "children" of all ages to develop their wills in the right way. His suggestions were given with love and with full understanding of each devotee's particular needs and nature. He seldom admonished a person twice; he would point out, once, some weakness in a disciple and then maintain silence about it.]

• • •

"It is difficult to be near a fragrant rose or an ill-odored skunk without being affected by it," the Master said. "So it is better to associate only with human roses."

• • •

"I like your teachings. But are you a Christian?" The questioner was talking for the first time with Paramahansaji. The Guru replied:

"Didn't Christ tell us: 'Not every one that

saith unto me, Lord, Lord, shall enter into the kingdom of heaven; but he that doeth the will of my Father which is in heaven'?"*

"In the Bible the term *heathen* means an idolater: one whose attention is centered not on the Lord but on the attractions of the world. A materialist may go to church on Sundays and still be a heathen. He who keeps ever alight the lamp of remembrance of the Heavenly Father and who obeys the precepts of Jesus is a Christian." He added, "It is for you to decide whether or not you think I am a Christian."

• • •

"You see how good it is to work for the Lord," the Master said to a willing and painstaking disciple. "The sense of egotism or selfishness within us is a test. Will we wisely labor for the Heavenly Father or foolishly for ourselves?

"By performing actions in the right spirit, we come to understand that the Lord is the only Doer; that is, all power is divine and flows from the Sole Being, God."

• • •

"Life is a great dream of God's," the Master said.

* Matthew 7:21.

"If it is only a dream, why is pain so real?" a student inquired.

"A dream head struck against a dream wall causes dream pain," Paramahansaji replied. "A dreamer is not cognizant of the hallucinatory fabric of a dream until he awakens. Similarly, man does not understand the delusory nature of the cosmic dream of creation until he awakens in God."

• • •

The Master stressed the need for a balanced life of activity and meditation.

"When you work for God, not self," he said, "it is just as good as meditation. Then work helps your meditation and meditation helps your work. You need the balance. With meditation only, you become lazy. With activity only, the mind becomes worldly and you forget God."

• • •

"It is beautiful to think that the Lord loves all of us equally," a visitor said, "but it seems unjust that He should care as much for a sinner as for a saint."

"Is a diamond less valuable because it is covered with mud?" the Master answered. "God sees the changeless beauty of our souls. He knows we are not our mistakes."

Many persons seem to defy progress, preferring well-worn ruts of thought and activity.

"I call such men 'psychological antiques,'" the Master said to the disciples. "Don't be one of them, lest when you die the angels say, 'Oh, here comes an antique! Let us send him back to earth!'"*

. . .

"What is the difference between a worldly person and an evil person?" a man asked. The Master said:

"Most men are worldly; few are really evil. 'Worldly' means being foolish, giving importance to trifling matters, and staying away from God out of ignorance. But 'evil' means deliberately turning one's back on the Lord; not many would do that."

. . .

A new student thought it possible to assimilate the Master's teachings through deep study alone, without practicing meditation. Paramahansaji told him:

"The perception of truth must be a growth from within. It cannot be a graft."

* See "reincarnation" in glossary.

"Do not lament if you see no lights or images in meditation," the Master told the devotees. "Go deep into the perception of Bliss; there you will find the actual presence of God. Seek not a part but the Whole."

•   •   •

A certain student, whom the Master had initiated in *Kriya Yoga,* said to another student:

"I don't practice *Kriya* daily. I am trying to retain the memory of the joy that came to me the first time I used the technique."

When Paramahansaji heard the story, he laughed and said:

"He is like a hungry man who refuses food, remarking: 'No, thanks. I am trying to hold on to the feeling of satisfaction I got from a meal last week.'"

•   •   •

"Master, I love everyone," a disciple said.

"You should love only God," Paramahansaji replied.

The disciple met the Guru a few weeks later. He asked her, "Do you love others?"

"I keep my love only for God," the devotee answered.

"You should love all with that same love."

The baffled disciple said, "Sir, what is your meaning? First you say that to love all is wrong; then you say that to exclude anyone is wrong."

"You are attracted to the personality of people; that leads to limiting attachments," the Master explained. "When you truly love God you will see Him in each face, and will know what it means to love all. It is not forms and egos we should adore, but the indwelling Lord in everyone. He alone informs His creatures with life, charm, and individuality."

•   •   •

A disciple expressed his desire to please the Master. Paramahansaji replied:

"My happiness lies in knowing that you are happy in God. Be anchored in Him."

•   •   •

"My desire for God is very intense," a disciple said. The Master replied:

"That is the greatest blessing, to feel His pull at your heart. It is His way of saying: 'Too long you have played with the toys of My creation. Now I want you with Me. Come home!'"

•   •   •

Some of the monks and nuns of the Self-Realization Order were discussing with Paramahansaji the relative merits of wearing monastic garb as a help in seeking God. The Master said:

"What matters is not your clothes but your attitude. Make your heart a hermitage, and your robe the love of God."

•   •   •

Discussing the folly of keeping bad company, the Master said, "Peeling garlic or touching a rotten egg leaves offensive smells on the hands, which then require a lot of washing."

•   •   •

"So long as we are immersed in body consciousness, we are like strangers in a foreign country," the Master said. "Our native land is Omnipresence."

•   •   •

A group of disciples were walking with the Master on the lawn of the Encinitas Hermitage, which overlooks the ocean. It was very foggy and dark. Someone remarked, "How cold and gloomy it is!"

"It is something like the atmosphere that envelops a materialistic person at the time of death," the Master said. "He slips from this world into what seems to be a heavy mist. Nothing is

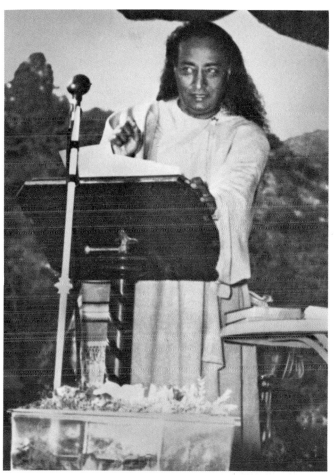

Paramahansa Yogananda speaking at dedication of Self-Realization Fellowship Lake Shrine and Gandhi World Peace Memorial, Pacific Palisades, California, 1950

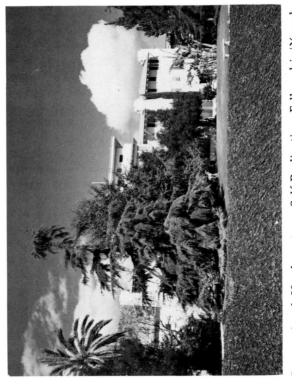

International Headquarters, Self-Realization Fellowship/Yogoda Satsanga Society of India; on Mt. Washington, Los Angeles, California clear to him; and for a time he feels lost and afraid. Then, in accordance with his karma, he either goes on to a bright astral world to learn spiritual lessons, or sinks into a stupor until the right karmic moment arrives for him to be reborn on earth.

"The consciousness of a devotee, one who loves God, is not disturbed by the transition from this world to the next. He effortlessly enters a realm of light, love, and joy."

•   •   •

"Most persons are engrossed in material things," the Master said. "If they think of God at all, it is only to ask Him for money or health. They seldom pray for the supreme gift: the sight of His face, the transforming touch of His hand.

"The Lord knows the course of our thoughts. He does not reveal Himself to us until we have surrendered to Him our last worldly desire; until each of us says: 'Father, guide and possess me.'"

•   •   •

"No matter which way you turn a compass, its needle points to the north," the Master said. "So it is with the true yogi. Immersed he may be in many outer activities, but his mind is always on the Lord. His heart constantly sings: 'My God, my God, most lovable of all!'"

"Do not expect a spiritual blossom every day in the garden of your life," the Master said to a group of disciples. "Have faith that the Lord to whom you have surrendered yourselves will bring you divine fulfillment at the proper time.

"You have already sown the seed of God-aspiration; water it with prayer and right actions. Remove the weeds of doubt, indecision, and lethargy. When sprouts of divine perceptions appear, tend them with devotional care. One morning you will behold the flower of Self-realization."

• • •

Paramahansaji was giving a discourse before a group of disciples. A certain devotee, seemingly intent upon the Guru's words, allowed his thoughts to stray. When the time came to say good-night, Paramahansaji remarked to him:

"The mind is like a horse; it is good to tie it lest it run away."

• • •

Many men and women, not comprehending spiritual truths, resist the help that a sage is eager to give them. They reject his counsel suspiciously. One day Paramahansaji sighed:

"People are so skillful in their ignorance!"

An earnest new student, expecting overnight results as if by magic, was disappointed to find that after a week's effort in meditation he could detect no sign of God's presence within.

"If you don't discover the pearl by one or two divings, don't blame the ocean; find fault with your diving," the Master said. "You haven't yet plunged deep enough."

• • •

"By the practice of meditation," the Master said, "you will find that you are carrying within your heart a portable paradise."

• • •

The Master was the meekest of the meek in many ways, but on suitable occasion he could be adamant. A certain disciple, having seen only the soft side of Paramahansaji, began to neglect his duties. The Guru upbraided him sharply. Seeing the amazement in the young man's eyes at this unexpected discipline, the Master said:

"When you forget the high purpose that brought you here, I remember my spiritual obligation to correct your faults."

The Guru stressed the need for complete sincerity with God. He said:

"The Lord cannot be bribed by the size of the congregation in a church or by its wealth or by well-planned sermons. God visits only the altars of hearts that are cleansed by tears of devotion and lighted with candles of love."

•   •   •

A devotee was distressed because fellow disciples seemed to be making greater spiritual progress than he. The Master said:

"You keep your eyes on the big platter instead of on your own dish, thinking of what you didn't get instead of what has been given you."

•   •   •

The Master often said of his large family of truth seekers:

"Divine Mother sent me all these souls that I might drink the nectar of Her love from chalices of many hearts."

•   •   •

Interested in the spread of the Guru's message, a certain disciple would exult whenever the attendance at the Self-Realization Temple in Hollywood was especially large. But Paramahansaji said:

"A shopkeeper notices carefully how many persons visit his store. I never think that way about our church. I enjoy 'crowds of souls,' as I often say; but my friendship is given unconditionally to all, whether or not they come here."

• • •

To a discouraged disciple the Master said:

"Don't be negative. Never say that you are not progressing. When you think: 'I can't find God,' you yourself have given that verdict. Nobody else is keeping the Lord away from you."

• • •

"Master, tell me the prayer I should use to draw to me most quickly the Divine Beloved," a Hindu devotee said. Paramahansaji replied:

"Give God the gems of prayer lying deep in the mine of your own heart."

• • •

The Master, always openhanded, ever giving away that which had been given to him, once said: "I don't believe in charity." Observing the amazement on the disciples' faces, he added:

"Charity enslaves people. To share your wisdom with others, so they are enabled to help themselves, is greater than any material gift."

•   •   •

"A bad habit can be quickly changed," the Master said to a disciple seeking his help.

"A habit is the result of concentration of the mind. You have been thinking in a certain way. To form a new and good habit, just concentrate in the opposite direction."

•   •   •

"When you have learned to be happy in the *present*, you have found the right path to God," the Master said to a group of disciples.

"Very few persons, then, are living in the present," a devotee observed.

"True," Paramahansaji replied. "Most are living in thoughts of the past or the future."

•   •   •

A student who had met many disappointments began to lose faith in God. To him the Master said:

"The moment when Divine Mother beats you the hardest is the time you should cling tenaciously to Her skirt."

Talking about the evils of gossip, the Master told a group of disciples:

"My guru Sri Yukteswar used to say: 'If it isn't something I may tell everybody, I don't want to hear it.'"

• • •

"The Lord brought into being both man and *maya*," the Master said. "The states of delusion—anger, greed, selfishness, and so on—are His inventions, not ours. He is responsible for planning the tests in the obstacle race of life.

"A great saint of India used to pray: 'Heavenly Father, I didn't ask to be created; but, since Thou hast created me, please release me in Thy Spirit.' If you lovingly speak to God in this way, He will have to take you Home."

• • •

"Do not be impressed by the praise of acquaintances who really do not know you," the Master said. "Rather seek the good opinion of true friends—those who help you to improve yourself and who never flatter you or condone your faults. It is God who is guiding you through the sincerity of real friends."

Two students came together to the Mt. Washington Center for training. The other devotees thought highly of them. In a short time, however, the two students left. The Master said to the ashram residents:

"You were impressed by their actions, but I was watching their thoughts. Inwardly they were running wild, though outwardly they followed all the rules. Good conduct will not last long if one does not adopt proper means to purify the mind."

• • •

A man was deeply attracted to Paramahansaji but would not follow his advice. The Master said:

"I cannot be displeased with him; for, though he makes many mistakes, his heart yearns for God. If he would let me, I would lead him quickly to the Divine Home; nevertheless, in time he will get there. He is a Cadillac stuck in the mud."

• • •

To a dissatisfied student, the Master said:

"Don't doubt, or God will remove you from the hermitage. So many come here looking for miracles. But masters do not display the powers

God has given them unless He commands them to do so. Most men don't understand that the greatest miracle of all would be the transformation of their lives by humble obedience to His will."

• • •

"God sent you here for a purpose," the Master said. "Are you acting in harmony with that purpose? You came on earth to accomplish a divine mission. Realize how tremendously important that is! Do not allow the narrow ego to obstruct your attainment of an infinite goal."

• • •

A disciple was excusing his lack of spiritual progress on the grounds that he had difficulty in overcoming his faults.

Intuitively perceiving a deeper cause, Paramahansaji said:

"The Lord doesn't mind your faults. He minds your indifference."

• • •

When the Master was leaving Boston in 1923, to start on a transcontinental tour to spread the Self-Realization Fellowship teachings, one of his students remarked:

"Sir, I shall feel helpless without your spiritual guidance." The Master replied:

"Don't depend on me. Depend on God."

•   •   •

To certain resident ashram disciples who often visited old friends on weekends, the Master said:

"You are becoming restless and wasting your time. You came here for God-realization and now you are cheating yourselves by forgetting your Goal. Why seek outside diversions? Find the Lord and see what you have been missing!"

•   •   •

Two young disciples were often in each other's company in the hermitage. The Master said to them:

"It is limiting to be attached to just one or only a few persons, excluding everyone else. Such a course inhibits the growth of universal sympathy. You should extend the boundaries of the kingdom of your affections. Scatter your love everywhere to the God in everything."

•   •   •

Looking at the stars while strolling one evening with a group of disciples, the Master said:

"Each of you is composed of many tiny stars —stars of atoms! If your life force were released from the ego, you would find yourself aware of the whole universe. When great devotees die, they feel their consciousness spreading over infinite space. It is a beautiful experience."

. . .

To the congregation of the Self-Realization Temple in San Diego, the Master said:
"Let the church remind you of your own cathedral within, where you should go in the dead of night and in the dawn. There you can listen to the mighty organ of music of *Aum* and hear in it the sermon of divine wisdom."

. . .

One evening as he sat talking with the disciples, the Master said:
"Possessions mean nothing to me, but friendship is very dear. In true companionship one catches a glimpse of the Friend of all Friends." After a pause, he continued, "Never be false to a friend or betray anyone. To do so is one of the greatest sins before the Divine Tribunal."

Paramahansaji was leaving the Mt. Washington Center to give a lecture, but he stopped for a few minutes to talk with one of the disciples. The Master said:

"It is a good idea to keep a mental diary. Before you go to bed each night, sit for a short time and review the day. See what you are becoming. Do you like the trend of your life? If not, change it."

• • •

A television set was given to the Master. It was set up in a room where it could be used by all the disciples. They were going there so frequently that the Master said to them:

"So long as you have not found God, it is best not to be interested in amusements. Seeking diversion means forgetting Him. First learn to love Him and know Him. Then it won't matter what you do, for He will never leave your thoughts."

• • •

"Indulgence in sense joys is followed by satiety and disgust," the Master said. "These constant dual experiences make man moody and unreliable. *Maya* or the state of delusion is characterized by the pairs of opposites. Through meditation on God, the Sole Unity, the devotee banishes from his mind the alternating waves of pleasure and pain."

. . .

"Master, when I am older and have seen more of life I shall renounce all and seek God. Right now there is too much I want to know and experience," a student said.

After he had departed from the hermitage, Paramahansaji remarked:

"He still believes that sex is love and that 'things' are wealth. He will become like the man whose wife had forsaken him and whose house had burned down. Reflecting on his losses, the man determined to 'give up all.' The Lord is not much impressed by such 'renunciation.' The student who has just abandoned his training here will not be willing to 'renounce all' until he has nothing material left to renounce!"

. . .

"It hardly seems practical to think about God all the time," a visitor remarked. The Master replied:

"The world agrees with you, and is the world a happy place? True joy eludes the man who forsakes God, because He is Bliss Itself. On earth His devotees live in an inner heaven of peace; but those who forget Him pass their days in a self-created hades of insecurity and disappointment. To 'make friends' with the Lord is to be really practical!"

•   •   •

Paramahansaji asked a certain disciple to do some work at a Self-Realization retreat in the desert. The devotee went reluctantly, worrying about duties he had left behind him at the Mt. Washington Center.

"Your new work at the desert retreat should be your only concern now," the Master told him. "Do not feel attachment to anything. Accept changes with equanimity, and perform in a spirit of divine freedom whatever duties come your way.

"If God were to say to me today: *Come home!* without a backward glance I would leave all my obligations here — organization, buildings, plans, people — and hasten to obey Him. Running the world is His responsibility. He is the Doer, not you or I."*

•   •   •

"Guruji," a disciple asked, "If you could set time back to the point where your Master asked you to undertake organizational work, would

* See "ego" in glossary.

you be glad to consent — knowing what you do now about the burden of responsibility for many other persons?" The Master replied:

"Yes, such work teaches unselfishness."

• • •

The age-old question of why God permits suffering was often put to Paramahansaji. Patiently he would explain:

"Suffering is caused by the misuse of free will. God has given us the power to accept Him or reject Him. He doesn't want us to encounter woes, but will not interfere when we choose actions that lead to misery.

"Men do not heed the wisdom of the saints, but expect unusual circumstances or miracles to save them when they get into trouble. The Lord can do anything; but He knows that man's love and right conduct cannot be bought with miracles.

"God has sent us out as His children, and in that divine role we must return to Him. The only way to reunion is through the exercise of your own will. No other power on earth or in heaven can do it for you. But when you give a real soul-call, God sends you a guru to lead you from the wilderness of pain to His home of eternal joy.

"The Lord has given you free will, and so He cannot act as a dictator. Although He is Almighty Power, He does not arrange that you be released

from suffering when you have chosen the path of
evil actions. Is it just to expect Him to remove
your burdens if your thoughts and deeds are op-
posed to His laws? In observance of His code of
ethics, such as He gave in the Ten Command-
ments, lies the secret of happiness."

• • •

Paramahansaji frequently warned disciples
of the dangers of spiritual idleness. "The minutes
are more important than the years," he would
say. "If you do not fill the minutes of your life
with thoughts of God, the years will slip by; and
when you need Him most you may be unable to
feel His presence. But if you fill the minutes of
your life with divine aspirations, automatically
the years will be saturated with them."

• • •

In ancient India the term *guru* applied only
to Christlike masters capable of conveying divine realization to disciples. Following the scriptural injunctions, the devotees made themselves
spiritually receptive through unquestioning
obedience to the training of the holy preceptor.
Westerners sometimes objected to such volun-
tary subjection of personal freedom to the will of
another, but the Master said:

"When one has found his guru there should

be unconditional devotion to him, because he is the vehicle of God. The guru's sole purpose is to bring the disciple to Self-realization; the love a guru receives from a devotee is given by the guru to God. When a spiritual preceptor finds a student in tune with him, he is able to teach him more quickly than he can teach a student who resists him.

"I am not your leader but your servant. I am as the dust at your feet. I see God represented in you, and I bow to you all. I want only to tell you of the great joy that I feel in Him. I have no personal ambition, but I have the greatest ambition to share my spiritual joy with all peoples of the earth."

•   •   •

In a talk to the ashram residents, Sri Yogananda said: "In the spiritual life one becomes just like a little child—without resentment, without attachment, full of life and joy. Let nothing hurt or disturb you. Be still within, receptive to the Divine Voice. Spend your leisure time in meditation.

"I have never known any pleasure of the world as great as the spiritual joy of *Kriya Yoga*. I would not give it up for all the comforts of the West or all the gold in the world. I have found it possible through *Kriya Yoga* to carry my happiness always with me."

The Master painted many unforgettable word-pictures to illustrate a spiritual point. "Life is like this," he once remarked. "You have prepared a picnic dinner and suddenly a bear comes and overturns the table and you are forced to run away. Men lead their lives in that way: they work for a little joy and security; then the bear of disease comes, their heart stops, and they are gone.

"Why live in such a state of uncertainty? Unimportant things in your life have assumed first place. You allow various activities to engage your time and enslave you. How many years have gone by in this manner? Why let the remainder of life slip by without spiritual progress? If you make up your mind today that you will not let obstacles deter you, you will be given the power to overcome them."

•   •   •

"A lazy person never finds God," the Master said. "An idle mind becomes the workshop of the devil. I have seen many *sannyasis* [monks] who renounced work and became nothing more than beggars. But persons who work for a living without any wish for the fruits of action, desiring the Lord alone, are true renunciants. It is very difficult to practice such renunciation, but when you so love God that everything you do is to please Him, you are free.

"In thinking: 'I am working only for God,'

your love becomes so great that you have no other thought in your mind, no other objective, but to serve and adore Him."

•   •   •

"Behold the altar of God in the stars, beneath the earth, and behind the throb of your feelings," the Master said. "He, the neglected Reality, is hidden everywhere. If you follow the path steadfastly and meditate regularly you will see Him in a golden robe of light that spreads throughout eternity. Behind each thought you will feel His blissful presence.

"God is not to be just talked about. Many have spoken about Him; many have wondered about Him; many have read about Him. But few have tasted His joy. Only those few know Him. And when you know Him, no longer do you stand aside and worship Him; you become one with Him. Then, as Jesus and all other masters have said, you too may say: 'I and my Father are one.'"

•   •   •

The Master said: "By diving deep through your spiritual eye* you will see into the fourth dimension,† aglow with the wonders of the inner

---

* See glossary.
† See "astral worlds" in glossary.

world. It is hard to get there, but how beautiful it is!

"Don't be satisfied with a little peace born of your meditation, but hunger again and again for His bliss. Day and night, while others are sleeping or spending their energy in fulfilling desires, you should whisper, 'My Lord, my Lord, my Lord!' And in time He will burst through the darkness and you will know Him. This world is an ugly place compared to the lovely realm of Spirit. Remove the obstacles to divine insight by determination, devotion, and faith."

• • •

"At Christmastime there are strong vibrations of Christ Consciousness in the air," the Master said. "Those who are attuned by their devotion and by deep, scientific meditation will receive the divine vibrations. It is of the utmost spiritual importance to every man, whatever his religion, that he experience within himself this 'birth' of the universal Christ.

"The cosmos is his body. Everywhere present within it is the Christ Consciousness. When you can close your eyes and by meditation expand your awareness until you feel the whole universe as your own body, Christ will have been born within you. All clouds of ignorance will be dispelled as you behold, behind the darkness of closed eyes, the divine cosmic light.

"Christ should be worshiped in truth: first in spirit, by meditation; and second in form, by perceiving his presence in even the material world. You should meditate on the real meaning of the coming of Christ, and feel his consciousness drawn within you by the magnet of your devotion. That is the real purpose of Christmas."

• • •

Balance is a key word in the teachings of Paramahansaji. "If you practice meditation deeply, your mind will turn more and more intensely toward God," he said. "However, you must not neglect your duties in the world. As you learn to perform all your tasks with a peaceful mind you will be able to do things more quickly, with greater concentration and efficiency. You will then find that no matter what you do, your activities will be permeated with the divine consciousness. That state comes only after you have practiced meditation deeply and disciplined your mind to revert to God as soon as you have performed your duties, and by doing them with the thought that you are serving Him alone."

• • •

"Repentance doesn't mean merely to be sorry for a misdoing but also to refrain from performing that act again," the Master said. "When you repent truly, you determine to forsake evil. The heart is often very hard; it is not easily moved. Soften it by prayer. Then divine blessing comes."

• • •

"Be guided by wisdom," the Master said. "Past wrong actions have left seeds in your mind. If you set the seeds afire by wisdom they become 'roasted' or ineffectual. You cannot achieve emancipation until you have burned the seeds of past actions in the fires of wisdom and meditation. If you want to destroy the bad effects of past actions, meditate. What you have done you can undo. If you are not growing spiritually, in spite of trials you must try and try again. When your present efforts become more powerful than the karma of past actions, you are free."

• • •

During a lecture Paramahansaji said: "Christ told each of us to 'love thy neighbor as thyself.' But without soul knowledge, by which you realize that all men are indeed 'thyself,' you cannot follow Christ's command. To me there is no difference among men, because I see each one as God's child. I can't think of anyone as a stranger.

"Once in New York City three holdup men

surrounded me. I said: 'Do you want money? Take it,' and held out my wallet. I was in the superconscious state. The men did not reach for the wallet. Finally one of them said:

"'Beg your pardon. We can't do it.' They ran away.

"On another night in New York, near Carnegie Hall where I had just delivered a lecture, a man with a gun approached me. He said:

"'Do you know I can shoot you?'

"'Why?' I asked calmly. My mind was on God.

"'You talk about democracy.' He was obviously a mentally disturbed person. We stood in silence for a while, then he said:

"'Forgive me. You have taken away my evil.' He ran down the street as swiftly as a stag.

"Those who are in tune with God can change men's hearts."

•   •   •

"To state that the world is a dream, without trying to attain in meditation actual realization of this truth, may lead one to fanaticism," the Master said. "The wise man understands that even though mortal life is a dream, it contains dream pains. He adopts scientific methods to awaken from the dream."

When the chapel at Self-Realization Fellowship headquarters was being redecorated, a disciple suggested that a niche hold a sanctuary lamp, known as a "perpetual candle," to be lit by Paramahansaji.

The Master said, "I would like to feel that the lamp of devotion to God I have lit in your hearts is eternal. No other light is necessary."

• • •

During 1951 Paramahansaji often hinted that his remaining days on earth were not many.

"Sir," asked a distressed disciple, "when we can no longer see you, will you be as near as you are now?"

The Master smiled lovingly and said:

"To those who think me near, I will be near."

PARAMAHANSA YOGANANDA:
A YOGI IN LIFE AND DEATH

Paramahansa Yogananda entered *mahasamadhi* (a yogi's final conscious exit from the body) in Los Angeles, California, on March 7, 1952, after concluding his speech at a banquet held in honor of H. E. Binay R. Sen, Ambassador of India.

The great world teacher demonstrated the value of yoga (scientific techniques for God-realization) not only in life but in death. Weeks after his departure his unchanged face shone with the divine luster of incorruptibility.

Mr. Harry T. Rowe, Los Angeles Mortuary Director, Forest Lawn Memorial-Park (in which the body of the great master is temporarily placed), sent Self-Realization Fellowship a notarized letter from which the following extracts are taken:

"The absence of any visual signs of decay in the dead body of Paramahansa Yogananda offers the most extraordinary case in our experience .... No physical disintegration was visible in his body even twenty days after death .... No indication of mold was visible on his skin, and no visible desiccation (drying up) took place in the bodily tissues. This state of perfect preservation of a body is, so far as we know from mortuary annals, an unparalleled one .... At the time of receiving Yogananda's body, the Mortuary personnel expected to observe, through the glass lid of the casket, the usual progressive signs of bodily decay. Our astonishment increased as day followed day without bringing any visible change in the body under observation. Yogananda's body was apparently in a phenomenal state of immutability ....

"No odor of decay emanated from his body at any time .... The physical appearance of Yogananda on March 27th, just before the bronze cover of the casket was put into position, was the same as it had been on March 7th. He looked on March 27th as fresh and as unravaged by decay as he had looked on the night of his death. On March 27th there was no reason to say that his body had suffered any visible physical disintegration at all. For these reasons we state again that the case of Paramahansa Yogananda is unique in our experience."

AIMS AND IDEALS
of
Self-Realization Fellowship

As set forth by Paramahansa Yogananda, Founder
Sri Daya Mata, President

To disseminate among the nations a knowledge of definite scientific techniques for attaining direct personal experience of God.

To teach that the purpose of life is the evolution, through self-effort, of man's limited mortal consciousness into God Consciousness; and to this end to establish Self-Realization Fellowship temples for God-communion throughout the world, and to encourage the establishment of individual temples of God in the homes and in the hearts of men.

To reveal the complete harmony and basic oneness of original Christianity as taught by Jesus Christ and original Yoga as taught by Bhagavan Krishna; and to show that these principles of truth are the common scientific foundation of all true religions.

To point out the one divine highway to which all paths of true religious beliefs eventually lead: the highway of daily, scientific, devotional meditation on God.

To liberate man from his threefold suffering: physical disease, mental inharmonies, and spiritual ignorance.

To encourage "plain living and high thinking"; and to spread a spirit of brotherhood among all peoples by teaching the eternal basis of their unity: kinship with God.

To demonstrate the superiority of mind over body, of soul over mind.

To overcome evil by good, sorrow by joy, cruelty by kindness, ignorance by wisdom.

To unite science and religion through realization of the unity of their underlying principles.

To advocate cultural and spiritual understanding between East and West, and the exchange of their finest distinctive features.

To serve mankind as one's larger Self.

GLOSSARY

Astral worlds: The beautiful realms of light and joy to which persons with a measure of spiritual understanding go for further development after death. Even higher is the causal or ideational sphere. These worlds are described in chapter 43 of *Autobiography of a Yogi*.

Aum or Om: The basis of all sounds; universal symbol-word for God. *Aum* of the Vedas *(q.v.)* became the sacred word *Hum* of the Tibetans; *Amin* of the Moslems, and *Amen* of the Egyptians, Greeks, Romans, Jews, and Christians. *Amen* in Hebrew means *sure, faithful*. *Aum* is the all-pervading sound emanating from the Holy Ghost (Invisible Cosmic Vibration; God in His aspect of Creator); the "Word" of the Bible; the voice of creation, testifying to the Divine Presence in every atom. *Aum* may be heard through practice of Self-Realization Fellowship methods of meditation.

"These things saith the Amen, the faithful and true witness, the beginning of the creation of God."—Revelation 3:14. "In the beginning was the Word, and the Word was with God, and the Word was God.... All things were made by him [the Word or *Aum*]; and without him was not any thing made that was made." — John 1:1–3.

Babaji: Guru of Lahiri Mahasaya (guru of Swami Sri Yukteswar, who in turn was the guru of Paramahansa Yogananda). Babaji is a deathless avatar, living secretly in the Himalayas. His title is *Mahavatar* or "Divine Incarnation." Glimpses of his Christlike life are given in Paramahansa Yogananda's *Autobiography of a Yogi*.

Bhagavad-Gita ("Song of the Lord"): The Hindu Bible: sacred sayings of Lord Krishna, compiled millenniums ago by the sage Vyasa. See *Krishna*.

breath: "The breath links man to creation," Yoganandaji

wrote. "The influx of innumerable cosmic currents into man by way of the breath induces restlessness in his mind. To escape from the ceaseless flux of the phenomenal worlds and enter the infinity of Spirit, the yogi learns to quiet the breath by scientific meditation."

Christ consciousness: Awareness of Spirit as immanent in every atom of vibratory creation.

cosmic consciousness: Awareness of Spirit as transcending finite creation.

delusion: See *maya*.

Divine Mother: "That aspect of the Uncreated Infinite which is active in creation is referred to in Hindu scriptures as the Divine Mother," Paramahansaji wrote. "It is this personalized aspect of the Absolute that may be said to have 'longings' for the rightful behavior of Her children and to answer their prayers. Men who imagine that the Impersonal cannot manifest in a personal form are in effect denying Its omnipotence and the possibility that man can commune with his Maker. The Lord in the form of the Cosmic Mother appears in living tangibility before true *bhaktas* (devotees of a Personal God).

"The Lord manifests Himself before His saints in whatever form each of them holds dear. A devout Christian sees Jesus; a Hindu beholds Krishna, or the Goddess Kali, or an expanding Light if his worship takes an impersonal turn."

ego: The ego-principle, *ahankara* (lit., "I do"), is the root cause of dualism or the seeming separation between man and his Creator. *Ahankara* brings human beings under the sway of *maya (q.v.)*, by which the subject (ego) falsely appears as object; the creatures imagine themselves to be creators.

By banishing ego-consciousness, man awakens to his divine identity, his oneness with the sole Life, God.

guru: The spiritual preceptor who introduces the disciple to God. The term "guru" differs from "teacher," as a person may have many teachers but can have only one guru.

Holy Ghost: See *Aum.*

intuition: The "sixth sense"; apprehension of knowledge derived immediately and spontaneously from the soul, not from the fallible agency of the senses or of reason.

ji: A suffix denoting respect that is often added to names in India. Paramahansa Yogananda is therefore occasionally referred to in this book as Paramahansaji or Yoganandaji.

Kali: Mythological Hindu Goddess, represented as a woman with four hands. One hand symbolizes Nature's creative powers; the second hand represents the cosmic preservative functions; the third hand is an emblem of the purifying forces of dissolution. Kali's fourth hand is out-stretched in a gesture of blessing and salvation. Through these means She calls all creation back to its divine Source. Goddess Kali is a symbol or aspect of the Divine Mother *(q.v.).*

karma: The equilibrating law of karma, as expounded in the Hindu scriptures, is that of action and reaction, cause and effect, sowing and reaping. In the course of natural righteousness, each man, by his thoughts and actions, becomes the molder of his destiny. Whatever energies he himself, wisely or unwisely, has set in motion must return to him as their starting point, like a circle inexorably completing itself. "The world looks like a mathematical equation, which, turn it how you will, balances itself. Every secret is told, every crime is punished, every virtue rewarded, every wrong redressed, in silence and certainty" (Emerson, in *Compensation*). An understanding of karma as the law of justice serves to free the human mind from resentment against God and man. See *Reincarnation.*

Krishna: (d. 3102 B.C.) An avatar of India whose divine counsel in the Bhagavad-Gita *(q.v.)* is revered by all God-seekers. In early life he was a cowherd who enchanted his companions with the music of his flute. Allegorically, Lord Krishna represents the soul playing the flute of meditation to guide all misled thoughts back to the fold of omniscience.

Kriya Yoga: An ancient science developed in India for the use of God-seekers. Its technique is referred to and praised by Krishna in the Bhagavad-Gita and by Patanjali in the *Yoga Sutras.* The liberating science, which leads the practitioner to the attainment of cosmic consciousness, is taught to SRF members.

Lahiri Mahasaya (1828–1895): Guru of Sri Yukteswar *(q.v.)*, and disciple of Babaji *(q.v.)*. Lahiri Mahasaya revived the ancient, almost-lost science of yoga, giving the name of *Kriya Yoga* to the practical techniques. He was a Christlike teacher with miraculous powers; he was also a family man with business responsibilities. His mission was to make known a yoga suitable for modern man, in which meditation is balanced by right performance of worldly duties. Lahiri Mahasaya was a *Yogavatar* or "Incarnation of Yoga."

maya: Cosmic delusion; literally, "the measurer." *Maya* is the magical power in creation by which limitations and divisions are apparently present in the Immeasurable and Inseparable.

Sri Yogananda wrote in *Autobiography of a Yogi:*

"It should not be imagined that the truth about *maya* was understood only by the *rishis* (Hindu sages). The Old Testament prophets called *maya* by the name of Satan (lit., in Hebrew, 'the adversary'). Satan or *Maya* is the Cosmic Magician who produces multiplicity of forms to hide the One Formless Verity. The sole purpose of Satan is to divert man from Spirit to matter. Christ described *maya* picturesquely as a devil, a murderer, and a liar. 'The devil....was a murderer from the beginning, and abode not in the truth, because there is no truth in him. When he speaketh a lie, he speaketh of his own: for he is a liar, and the father of it' (John 8:44)."

Mount Washington Center: International headquarters of Self-Realization Fellowship (Yogoda Satsanga Society of India), established in Los Angeles in 1925 by Paramahansa Yogananda. The hilltop site, overlooking the heart of Los Angeles, covers seventeen acres. In the main administration building (see photo facing p. 71), the rooms of Gurudeva Paramahansa Yogananda are maintained as a shrine. From this Mother Center, Self-Realization Fellowship distributes the teachings of Paramahansaji in printed lesson form to members, and publishes his other writings and talks through numerous books and the quarterly magazine, *Self-Realization*.

nirbikalpa samadhi: The highest or irrevocably God-united stage of *samadhi*. The first or preliminary stage (characterized by trance, bodily immobility) is called *sabikalpa samadhi*.

Paramahansa: A religious title, signifying one who is master of himself. It is bestowed on a disciple by his guru. *Paramahansa* literally means "supreme swan." The swan is referred to in Hindu scriptures as a symbol of spiritual discrimination.

reincarnation: The doctrine, expounded in the Hindu scriptures, that man is born again and again on this earth. The cycle of reincarnation ceases when man consciously regains his status as a son of God. "Him that overcometh will I make a pillar in the temple of my God, and he shall go no more out." — Rev. 3:12. Understanding of the law of karma and of its corollary, reincarnation, is implicit in many Biblical passages.

The early Christian church accepted the doctrine of reincarnation, which was expounded by the Gnostics and by numerous church fathers, including Clement of Alexandria, the celebrated Origen, and the fifth-century St. Jerome. The theory was first declared a heresy in A.D. 553 by the Second Council of Constantinople. At that time many Christians thought the doctrine of reincarnation afforded man too ample a stage of time and space to encourage him to strive for immediate salvation. Today many Western thinkers accept the theories of karma and reincarnation, seeing in them the laws of justice that underlie life's seeming inequalities. See *karma*.

sadhu: One who pursues a *sadhana* or path of spiritual discipline; an ascetic.

samadhi: Superconsciousness. *Samadhi* is attained by following the eightfold yoga path, in which *samadhi* is the eighth step or final goal. Scientific meditation—the right use of yoga techniques anciently developed by India's sages —leads the devotee to *samadhi* or God-realization. Just as the wave melts in the sea, so the human soul realizes itself as omnipresent Spirit.

Sat-Tat-Aum: Father, Son, and Holy Ghost; or, God as transcendent or *nirguna*, "without qualities" — Cosmic Consciousness in the blissful void beyond the phenomenal worlds; God as Christ Consciousness, immanent in creation; and God as *Aum (q.v.)*, the Divine Creative Vibration.

Self-Realization Fellowship (SRF): A nonprofit, nonsectarian religious and educational organization, founded in America in 1920 by Paramahansa Yogananda. Its affiliate in India is Yogoda Satsanga Society (YSS), founded in 1917 by Paramahansa Yogananda.

spiritual eye: The "single" eye of wisdom, the pranic star door through which man must enter to attain cosmic consciousness. The method of entering the sacred door is taught to members of Self-Realization Fellowship.

"I am the door: by me if any man enter in, he shall be saved, and shall go in and out, and find pasture."—John 10:9. "When thine eye is single, thy whole body also is full of light.... Take heed, therefore, that the light which is in thee be not darkness." — Luke 11:34–35.

SRF Lessons: Compilations of the teachings of Paramahansa Yogananda, sent weekly to Self-Realization Fellowship members and students.

Self-Realization Order: The monastic Self-Realization Order founded by Paramahansa Yogananda. After a suitable period of training, eligible devotees may become monks and nuns of the Order. They take vows of simplicity (nonattachment to possessions), celibacy, obedience (willingness to follow the rules of life outlined by Paramahansa Yogananda), and loyalty (dedication to serving Self-Realization Fellowship, the society founded by Paramahansa Yogananda). Through succession from Paramahansaji, who was a member of the Giri branch of the ancient Hindu monastic order founded by Swami Shankaracharya, monks and nuns of the Self-Realization Order who take their final vows belong also to the ancient Shankara order. (See "Swami.")

Sri Yukteswar (1855–1936): The great guru of Paramahansa Yogananda, who called his teacher *Jnanavatar* or "Incarnation of Wisdom."

swami: A member of India's most ancient monastic order, reorganized in the eighth century by Swami Shankaracharya. A swami takes formal vows of celibacy and renunciation of worldly ambitions; he devotes himself to meditation and service to humanity. There are ten classificatory titles attached to the Swami Order, as *Giri, Puri, Bharati, Tirtha, Saraswati,* and others. Swami Sri Yukteswar *(q.v.)* and Paramahansa Yogananda belonged to the *Giri* ("mountain") branch.

Vedas: The four scriptural texts of the Hindus: *Rig Veda, Sama Veda, Yajur Veda,* and *Atharva Veda.* They are essentially a literature of chant and recitation. Among the immense texts of India, the Vedas (from Sanskrit root *vid,* to know) are the only writings to which no author is ascribed. The *Rig*

Veda assigns a celestial origin to the hymns and tells us they have come down from "ancient times," reclothed in new language. Divinely revealed from age to age to the *rishis*, "seers," the Vedas are said to possess *nityatva*, "timeless finality."

yoga: Literally, "union" of man with his Maker through practice of scientific techniques for Self-realization. The three main paths are *Jnana Yoga* (wisdom), *Bhakti Yoga* (devotion), and *Raja Yoga* (the "royal" or scientific path, which includes the techniques of *Kriya Yoga*). The oldest text extant on the sacred science is Patanjali's *Yoga Sutras*. Patanjali's date is unknown, though some scholars assign him to the second century B.C.

yogi: One who practices yoga. He need not be a man of formal renunciation; a yogi is concerned solely with faithful daily practice of scientific techniques for God-realization.

Yogananda: The monastic name of Yogananda is a combination of two words, and means "bliss *(ananda)* through divine union *(yoga)*."

INDEX